EXAMINING SPECIAL NUTRITIONAL REQUIREMENTS

IN DISEASE STATES

PROCEEDINGS OF A WORKSHOP

Anne Brown Rodgers, *Rapporteur*

Food and Nutrition Board

Health and Medicine Division

The National Academies of
SCIENCES · ENGINEERING · MEDICINE

THE NATIONAL ACADEMIES PRESS
Washington, DC
www.nap.edu

THE NATIONAL ACADEMIES PRESS 500 Fifth Street, NW Washington, DC 20001

This activity was supported by contracts between the National Academy of Sciences and the Academy of Nutrition and Dietetics; American Society for Nutrition; Crohn's & Colitis Foundation; Health Canada; National Institutes of Health; and U.S. Food and Drug Administration. Any opinions, findings, conclusions, or recommendations expressed in this publication do not necessarily reflect the views of any organization or agency that provided support for the project.

International Standard Book Number-13: 978-0-309-47837-3
International Standard Book Number-10: 0-309-47837-5
Digital Object Identifier: https://doi.org/10.17226/25164

Additional copies of this publication are available from the National Academies Press, 500 Fifth Street, NW, Keck 360, Washington, DC 20001; (800) 624-6242 or (202) 334-3313; http://www.nap.edu.

Copyright 2018 by the National Academy of Sciences. All rights reserved.

Printed in the United States of America

Suggested citation: National Academies of Sciences, Engineering, and Medicine. 2018. *Examining special nutritional requirements in disease states: Proceedings of a workshop*. Washington, DC: The National Academies Press. doi: https://doi.org/10.17226/25164.

The National Academies of
SCIENCES · ENGINEERING · MEDICINE

The **National Academy of Sciences** was established in 1863 by an Act of Congress, signed by President Lincoln, as a private, nongovernmental institution to advise the nation on issues related to science and technology. Members are elected by their peers for outstanding contributions to research. Dr. Marcia McNutt is president.

The **National Academy of Engineering** was established in 1964 under the charter of the National Academy of Sciences to bring the practices of engineering to advising the nation. Members are elected by their peers for extraordinary contributions to engineering. Dr. C. D. Mote, Jr., is president.

The **National Academy of Medicine** (formerly the Institute of Medicine) was established in 1970 under the charter of the National Academy of Sciences to advise the nation on medical and health issues. Members are elected by their peers for distinguished contributions to medicine and health. Dr. Victor J. Dzau is president.

The three Academies work together as the **National Academies of Sciences, Engineering, and Medicine** to provide independent, objective analysis and advice to the nation and conduct other activities to solve complex problems and inform public policy decisions. The National Academies also encourage education and research, recognize outstanding contributions to knowledge, and increase public understanding in matters of science, engineering, and medicine.

Learn more about the National Academies of Sciences, Engineering, and Medicine at **www.nationalacademies.org**.

The National Academies of
SCIENCES · ENGINEERING · MEDICINE

Consensus Study Reports published by the National Academies of Sciences, Engineering, and Medicine document the evidence-based consensus on the study's statement of task by an authoring committee of experts. Reports typically include findings, conclusions, and recommendations based on information gathered by the committee and the committee's deliberations. Each report has been subjected to a rigorous and independent peer-review process and it represents the position of the National Academies on the statement of task.

Proceedings published by the National Academies of Sciences, Engineering, and Medicine chronicle the presentations and discussions at a workshop, symposium, or other event convened by the National Academies. The statements and opinions contained in proceedings are those of the participants and are not endorsed by other participants, the planning committee, or the National Academies.

For information about other products and activities of the National Academies, please visit www.nationalacademies.org/about/whatwedo.

PLANNING COMMITTEE ON EXAMINING SPECIAL NUTRITIONAL REQUIREMENTS FOR DISEASE STATES—A WORKSHOP[1]

BARBARA O. SCHNEEMAN (*Chair*), Professor Emerita, University of California, Davis

PATSY M. BRANNON, Professor, Division of Nutritional Sciences, Cornell University, Ithaca, NY

STEVEN K. CLINTON, Professor, Department of Internal Medicine, Division of Medical Oncology, The Ohio State University, Columbus

ALEX R. KEMPER, Chief of the Division of Ambulatory Pediatrics, Nationwide Children's Hospital, Columbus, OH

ERIN MACLEOD, Director of Metabolic Nutrition, Division of Genetics and Metabolism, Children's National Health System, Washington, DC

BERNADETTE P. MARRIOTT, Professor, Division of Gastroenterology and Hepatology, Department of Medicine, and Professor, Military Division, Department of Psychiatry, Medical University of South Carolina, Charleston

PATRICK J. STOVER, Vice Chancellor and Dean for Agriculture and Life Sciences at Texas A&M AgriLife, College Station

DAVID L. SUSKIND, Professor of Pediatrics, Division of Gastroenterology, Seattle Children's Hospital, Washington

GARY D. WU, Ferdinand G. Weisbrod Professor in Gastroenterology, Perelman School of Medicine, University of Pennsylvania, Philadelphia

Health and Medicine Division Staff

MARIA ORIA, Study Director
ALICE VOROSMARTI, Research Associate
CYPRESS LYNX, Senior Program Assistant
ANN L. YAKTINE, Director, Food and Nutrition Board

---

[1] The National Academies of Sciences, Engineering, and Medicine's planning committees are solely responsible for organizing the workshop, identifying topics, and choosing speakers. The responsibility for the published Proceedings of a Workshop rests with the workshop rapporteur and the National Academies.

Reviewers

This Proceedings of a Workshop was reviewed in draft form by individuals chosen for their diverse perspectives and technical expertise. The purpose of this independent review is to provide candid and critical comments that will assist the National Academies of Sciences, Engineering, and Medicine in making each published proceedings as sound as possible and to ensure that it meets the institutional standards for quality, objectivity, evidence, and responsiveness to the charge. The review comments and draft manuscript remain confidential to protect the integrity of the process.

We thank the following individuals for their review of this proceedings:

JOHN W. ERDMAN, Emeritus, University of Illinois at
    Urbana-Champaign
DENISE M. NEY, University of Wisconsin–Madison
ROBERT M. RUSSELL, Emeritus, Tufts University School of
    Medicine
DAVID L. SUSKIND, Seattle Children's Hospital

Although the reviewers listed above provided many constructive comments and suggestions, they were not asked to endorse the content of the proceedings nor did they see the final draft before its release. The review of this proceedings was overseen by **A. CATHERINE ROSS,** The Pennsylvania State University. She was responsible for making certain that an independent examination of this proceedings was carried out in accordance with standards of the National Academies and that all review comments were carefully considered. Responsibility for the final content rests entirely with the rapporteur and the National Academies.

Contents

APPENDIXES

Boxes, Figures, and Tables

TABLES

Acronyms and Abbreviations

AI   Adequate Intake
AND   Academy of Nutrition and Dietetics
ASN   American Society for Nutrition
ATP   adenosine triphosphate

BBB   blood–brain barrier
BMI   body mass index
BOND   Biomarkers of Nutrition for Development
BRINDA   Biomarkers Reflecting Inflammation and Nutritional
                Determinants of Anemia

CF   cystic fibrosis
CFD   cerebral folate deficiency
CFTR   cystic fibrosis transmembrane conductance regulator
CHOP   Children's Hospital of Pennsylvania
CKD   chronic kidney disease
CRP   C-reactive protein
CSF   cerebrospinal fluid

DHA   docosahexaenoic acid
DNA   deoxyribonucleic acid
DoD   Department of Defense
DRI   Dietary Reference Intake

EAR	Estimated Average Requirement
EEN	exclusive enteral nutrition
EPA	eicosapentaenoic acid

FARMM	Food and Resulting Microbial Metabolites
FDA	U.S. Food and Drug Administration
FODMAP	fermentable oligosaccharides, disaccharides, monosaccharides, and polyols

GFR	glomerular filtration rate
GI	gastrointestinal
GMP	glycomacropeptide
GRADE	Grading of Recommendations Assessment, Development and Evaluation

| IBD | inflammatory bowel disease |
| IOM | Institute of Medicine |

| MELAS | mitochondrial encephalopathy, lactic acidosis, and stroke-like episodes |
| MMA | methylmalonic aciduria |

NAD+	nicotinamide adenine dinucleotide
NADH	nicotinamide adenine dinucleotide + hydrogen
NADPH	nicotinamide adenine dinucleotide phosphate
NHANES	National Health and Nutrition Examination Survey
NIH	National Institutes of Health
NOS	nitric oxide synthase

PAH	phenylalanine hydroxylase
PEW	protein energy wasting
Phe	phenylalanine
PICO	Population, Intervention, Comparisons, Outcomes
PKU	phenylketonuria
PLP	pyridoxal phosphate

RCT	randomized controlled trial
RD	registered dietitian
RDA	Recommended Dietary Allowance

| TBI | traumatic brain injury |

UL   Tolerable Upper Intake Level

WCRF-AICR   World Cancer Research Fund and the American Institute
            for Cancer Research
WHO   World Health Organization

1

Introduction and Workshop Overview

On April 2–3, 2018, the Food and Nutrition Board of the National Academies of Sciences, Engineering, and Medicine convened a Workshop on Examining Special Nutritional Requirements in Disease States in Washington, DC.[1] As guided by the Statement of Task (see Box 1-1), the workshop had the following objectives:

- Examine pathophysiological mechanisms by which specific diseases impact nutrient metabolism and nutrition status and whether this impact would result in nutrient requirements that differ from the Dietary Reference Intakes (DRIs).
  - o Explore the role of genetic variation in nutrition requirements.
  - o Examine nutrient requirements in certain chronic conditions or acute phases for which emerging data suggest a contribution of nutrition status to disease outcomes. Consider the scientific evidence needed to establish such relationships and discuss principles about the relationship between nutrition requirements and specific diseases.

---

[1] The role of the workshop's planning committee was limited to planning the workshop, and this Proceedings of a Workshop was prepared by the workshop rapporteur as a factual summary of what occurred at the workshop. Statements, recommendations, and opinions expressed are those of individual presenters and participants and are not necessarily endorsed or verified by the National Academies of Sciences, Engineering, and Medicine, and they should not be construed as reflecting any group consensus.

BOX 1-1
Statement of Task

The National Academies proposes to convene a public workshop to explore the evidence for special nutritional requirements in disease states and medical conditions that cannot be met with a normal diet. The workshop will explore how these requirements may apply to the management of acute or chronic conditions or diseases that include inborn errors of metabolism, burns or surgical trauma, cancer, inflammatory bowel disease, traumatic brain injury, and other noncommunicable diseases or medical conditions. The workshop will review the currently available evidence used to determine potential nutritional requirements that are not encompassed within the normal population variation. The workshop discussions will also encompass the strengths and limitations of different types of evidence (e.g., clinical, non-clinical) in establishing whether special nutritional requirements exist for a given disease or medical condition and in establishing the safety and efficacy of such therapies.

Potential questions that may be addressed in the workshop include the following:

1. When does a physiological state result in a unique nutritional requirement? What principles identify disease-related nutritional requirements, i.e., requirements that are not encompassed within the normal population variation? When are genetic variations that impact a nutrient requirement within the framework of population variation and when are they sufficiently distinct?
2. What principles have been learned from the use of dietary/nutritional management of certain chronic diseases or conditions (e.g., inborn errors of metabolism)? Can those principles be expanded to cover other chronic conditions, such as inflammatory bowel disease? Can those principles be expanded to other situations in which an acute phase presents a special nutritional requirement, such as burns or traumatic brain injury? What are the barriers to nutritional management of these particular conditions?
3. How does a disease state impact nutrient metabolism and nutritional status? Conversely, what is the impact of nutritional status on the disease state? Are there markers of nutrient status/metabolism in a disease state? If nutritional status or nutrient metabolism modifies or is modified by a disease state, does this result in a related nutritional requirement?
4. How can nutritional interventions (meeting the nutritional requirements related to a disease state) improve patient outcomes?
5. What strategies currently exist to improve access to up-to-date disease management strategies and solutions?

o Explore how a disease state impacts nutrient metabolism and nutrition status and, conversely, what is the impact of nutrition status on the disease state.

- Identify promising approaches and challenges to establishing a framework for determining special nutrient requirements related to managing disease states.

During the planning phase of the workshop, the committee gave the presenters several broad questions about the topic of special nutrient requirements to consider as they developed their presentations:

1. What are the genetic basis and the related biological mechanism(s) that are disturbed in this specific disease state and how do they lead to the special nutritional requirement (or requirement for specific method of nutrient delivery)?
2. How well does the genetic make-up predict what the specific nutrient needs are for this disease state? What is the evidence that there is a nutritional requirement different from that of the healthy population? (Focus on specific nutrient[s], not diet as a whole.)
3. Is the disease state (or nutrition status or health-related outcomes) responsive to a specific nutritional intervention?
4. What are potential complexities, including heterogeneity of responses? Why do these heterogeneities occur?
5. Does a dose–response relationship exist between the nutrient and outcome of interest?
6. What are the gaps in information? Are there pressing research issues?

In guiding the presenters to consider these questions in relation to their particular disease specialty, the committee hoped to generate insights that would inform the discussions about the topic as a whole. This Proceedings of a Workshop summarizes the presentations and discussions that took place over the course of the workshop.[2] It is not intended to be a comprehensive summary of the topic. Furthermore, citations listed in the proceedings correspond to those presented on speakers' slides and explicitly referred to during discussions and do not constitute a comprehensive reference list on any of the subjects covered during the workshop.

---

[2] Materials from the workshop, including presentations and videos, can be found at http:// www.nationalacademies.org/hmd/Activities/Nutrition/ExaminingSpecialNutritional RequirementsinDiseaseStatesWorkshop/2018-APR-02.aspx (accessed June 14, 2018).

ORGANIZATION OF THIS PROCEEDINGS OF A WORKSHOP

The organization of this Proceedings of a Workshop parallels the workshop agenda. This chapter provides an overview of the objectives and scope of the workshop, along with welcoming and opening remarks. Speakers during this session also provided some background and context for later sessions by defining special nutrient requirements and describing underlying biological processes of special nutrient requirements. Chapter 2 summarizes Session 2 presentations and discussions. Speakers discussed nutrient needs due to loss of function in several genetic diseases, including phenylketonuria (PKU) hydroxylase deficiency, mitochondrial-associated metabolic disorders, and complex inborn errors of metabolism. Chapter 3 summarizes Session 3 presentations, which looked at nutrient needs resulting from disease-induced loss of function. Speakers discussed intestinal failure, cystic fibrosis, inflammatory bowel disease, blood–brain barrier dysfunction, and chronic kidney disease. Chapter 4 summarizes Session 4 presentations on disease-induced nutrient deficiencies and conditionally essential nutrients. The session focused on arginine in sickle cell anemia, potential nutrient needs in traumatic brain injury, and metabolic turnover, inflammation, and redistribution. This session was also to have included a presentation on nutrient needs in burns, cachexia, and surgery, but the presenter, Paul Wischmeyer of Duke University School of Medicine, was unable to participate. Chapter 5 summarizes Session 5 presentations, which considered a range of research issues that are relevant to building the evidence base in this area. Speakers discussed inflammatory bowel disease and cancer as illustrative examples. Chapter 6 summarizes the final session, in which a panel of presenters and participants were invited to reflect on themes and principles that emerged during the workshop and to discuss potential opportunities for progress in this area. The workshop closed with remarks by a speaker from each of the workshop sponsors. The speakers expressed their appreciation for the thoughtful presentations and discussions and highlighted key themes from the workshop that echo their own missions and initiatives. The workshop agenda is presented in Appendix A. Biographical sketches of the speakers and moderators are presented in Appendix B.

WELCOMING REMARKS

Barbara Schneeman, Professor Emerita, University of California, Davis, and chair of the Planning Committee, opened the workshop by providing background and insight on the origins of the workshop and the planning committee's approach to developing the agenda. She began by highlighting several key sentences from the Statement of Task, which captured the essence of the workshop's intent: The task is to convene a public workshop to explore the evidence for special nutritional requirements in disease states and medical conditions that cannot be met with normal diet. The workshop will review the currently available evidence used to determine potential nutritional requirements that are not encompassed within the normal population variation.

Schneeman then reviewed the five questions in the Statement of Task and pointed out that the Statement of Task did not cover medical foods. Medical foods are under the purview of the U.S. Food and Drug Administration (FDA), which has provided guidance on the criteria that are necessary for a product to be considered a medical food. The focus of this workshop, she emphasized, was on special nutrient requirements that would not be met through normal diets. Schneeman also noted that health claims, nutrient content claims, and structure and function claims attached to foods for the general population were not part of the workshop's task.

Schneeman then reviewed the workshop objectives, putting them in the context of related National Academies work, including the DRI reports, the 2017 consensus study report *Guiding Principles for Developing Dietary Reference Intakes Based on Chronic Disease* (NASEM, 2017a) and the 2018 proceedings *Nutrigenomics and the Future of Nutrition: Proceedings of a Workshop—in Brief* (NASEM, 2018).

Finally, Schneeman referred participants to the National Academies' report *Redesigning the Process for Establishing the* Dietary Guidelines for Americans (NASEM, 2017b). She noted that this report acknowledged that the *Dietary Guidelines for Americans* cover the general population, which may include individuals with certain types of chronic disease. All these reports together, she said, provide a useful framework for understanding the current thinking about nutrition for the general population. One of the questions left unresolved, however, Schneeman felt, is the role of nutrition in managing disease, which the current workshop would begin to explore.

With that context, Schneeman introduced the two speakers for this session. Patsy Brannon, Professor, Division of Nutritional Sciences, Cornell University, set the stage by providing an overview of DRIs and how special nutrient requirements might differ from them. Patrick Stover, Vice Chancellor and Dean for Agriculture and Life Sciences at Texas A&M AgriLife, discussed the underlying biological processes of special nutritional requirements, with a focus on biomarkers.

WHAT DEFINES A SPECIAL NUTRITIONAL REQUIREMENT?[3]

The traditional DRIs reflect a distribution of requirements and risk of adverse outcomes in a healthy population[4] (see Figure 1-1), although questions and controversies exist about what constitutes healthy when the general population contains a substantive prevalence of chronic disease. In this distribution, Brannon explained, the risk of adverse outcomes increases when intakes are too low or too high. The Estimated Average Requirement (EAR) is defined as the intake that meets the needs of 50 percent of the population, and the Tolerable Upper Intake Level (UL) is defined as a level of intake that, if consumed on a chronic basis, may lead to adverse outcomes. The Recommended Dietary Allowance (RDA) is set to meet the needs of 97.5 percent of the population.

Within this framework, intakes at or above the RDA and below the UL constitute an adequate and safe intake for healthy populations. Brannon noted that another way of looking at this distribution is the U-shaped curve nested within the distribution, which shows the EAR. Brannon then explained that the current process for setting DRIs occurs within a risk assessment framework. The first step is to identify one or more health outcome(s) related to consumption of a specific nutrient; causality is important in this relationship. Once a health outcome(s) is identified, the next step is to assess the dose–response association in order to set the reference value. Additional steps in the DRI process are to examine the assessment of intakes in the population and to characterize risk at various levels of intake.

Identifying Health Outcomes

Beginning in 1997, Brannon stated, the usual health outcome for DRIs was nutrient deficiency diseases, and most of the DRIs were set to prevent deficiency. Chronic disease endpoints were considered in setting DRIs for two nutrients—fiber and vitamin D. In 2011, beginning with vitamin D and calcium, DRI committees began to incorporate systematic reviews into their work. Regardless of the nutrient under consideration, DRI committees face a number of challenges in conducting these systematic reviews, including

- selecting outcomes with the greatest value; which may be a challenge of particular importance for special nutrient requirements because the health outcome for a specific disease population may differ from that of the healthy population;

---

[3] This section summarizes information presented by Patsy Brannon.

[4] For DRI values, see http://nationalacademies.org/HMD/Activities/Nutrition/SummaryDRIs/DRI-Tables.aspx (accessed June 6, 2018).

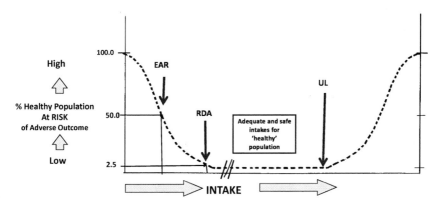

FIGURE 1-1 Traditional DRIs: distribution of requirement and risk of adverse outcome in a "healthy" population.
NOTE: DRI = Dietary Reference Intake; EAR = Estimated Average Requirement; RDA = Recommended Dietary Allowance; UL = Tolerable Upper Intake Level.
SOURCE: As presented by Patsy Brannon, April 2, 2018.

- identifying which outcomes, designs, populations, and other factors are of limited value;
- minimizing the differences in priorities and outlooks of the various members of the systematic review technical expert panel, which may affect decisions about the outcomes chosen;
- establishing instructions on weighing outcomes to eliminate variability; and
- selecting tools (e.g., evidence maps) to facilitate decision making.

The EAR and the RDA are usually based on the same health outcome because the EAR is specified, if possible, and then the RDA is set at two standard deviations above the EAR. When the existing evidence does not allow for the establishment of an EAR, an Adequate Intake (AI) is established. It is not certain as to how the AI relates to the distribution of the requirement, but it generally meets the needs of most of the population. The UL is often based on a different health outcome than the EAR and the RDA. Compared to the EARs and RDAs, a more cautious approach is taken in looking at the evidence for establishing ULs because randomized controlled trials (RCTs) are not typically conducted to identify toxicity health outcomes and, therefore, causality can be difficult to establish.

Nutritional Kinetics, Dynamics, and Requirements

Brannon noted that when nutrients are consumed, kinetic and dynamic processes occur that result in nutrient concentration at a site of action. At a minimum, the kinetic processes include absorption, which includes digestion and bioavailability, distribution in terms of the volume and the compartments in which the nutrient is distributed, metabolism, and excretion. The dynamic processes include actions, including toxicological actions, of the nutrient at a site in the body. These relate to dose response and effect, maximal efficacy, and the temporal response. Individuals vary in these kinetic and dynamic processes because of a number of factors, including genetics, epigenetics, age, sex, the physiological state (e.g., whether the individual is growing, pregnant, lactating), nutrient–diet interactions, nutrient–environment interactions, and drug–nutrient interactions. With this context, Brannon then noted that disease state is a critical factor that can affect the kinetics and dynamics of nutritional requirements. The following are several examples of how the nutritional requirements of several disease populations might differ from the distribution of nutrient need in a generally healthy population:

- Because of an alteration in phenylalanine metabolism, individuals with PKU may have a lower UL for ingestion of phenylalanine, relative to the distribution in a healthy population.
- Because of an impairment in digestion, most individuals with cystic fibrosis have an increased need for fat-soluble vitamins.

Special nutrition requirements can be thought of as a distribution of nutritional requirements for a specific disease population outside of the DRI distribution for healthy populations (see Box 1-2). The evidence needed to determine whether this difference exists would need to consider the following factors:

- The mechanism for the altered requirement. Is it kinetic, dynamic, system wide, tissue specific, or some combination thereof?
- Biomarkers of effect. What are the challenges of using biomarkers? Are systemic biomarkers or specific tissue biomarkers needed?

Brannon noted that the first step in setting DRIs—identifying the health outcome—helps determine whether the focus should be on management or nutritional treatment of the disease. The second step—determining dose–response—allows for a comparison to the DRI distribution for generally healthy populations so that a difference (if one exists) can be demonstrated.

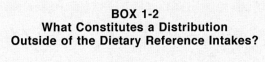

BOX 1-2
What Constitutes a Distribution
Outside of the Dietary Reference Intakes?

Disease with increased average nutritional requirement?

Disease with distribution shifted outside of DRI distribution?

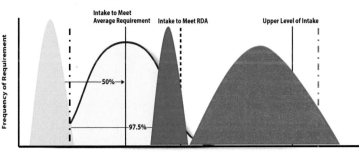

This graph, which shows a hypothetical nutrient requirement distribution for a population with a disease compared to the distribution of the same nutrient in the healthy population, illustrates three possibilities for a distribution outside of the DRIs: (1) The distribution in green might fall within the DRI, and, in that case, it would not necessarily constitute a special nutritional requirement; (2) The distribution in red shows a higher nutrient requirement distribution, potentially requiring a nutritional reference value higher than the recommended dietary allowance for the healthy population; (3) The distribution in yellow shows a lower nutrient requirement distribution, potentially requiring a lower nutritional reference value than the recommended dietary allowance for the healthy population.

NOTE: DRI = Dietary Reference Intake; RDA = Recommended Dietary Allowance
SOURCE: As presented by Patsy Brannon, April 2, 2018.

Brannon closed her remarks by stating that a particular challenge in the DRI-setting process is determining how to compare the distribution of a dose response for a special nutritional requirement if the health outcome for that disease population is a different health outcome than for the generally healthy population. She expressed the hope that workshop discussions would shed light on this issue.

THE UNDERLYING BIOLOGICAL PROCESSES OF
SPECIAL NUTRITIONAL REQUIREMENTS[5]

A central question that has been asked for years when considering recommendations about dietary and nutrient adequacy is adequate for what? The discussion around this question, Stover said, has evolved over time from an emphasis on avoiding deficiency to an emphasis on chronic disease prevention. The workshop's focus has taken this discussion a step further by considering disease management.

Stover then noted that the recent reports from the National Academies on the redesign process for the *Dietary Guidelines for Americans* (NASEM, 2017b) and the development of DRIs based on chronic diseases (NASEM, 2017a) are an acknowledgment that dietary recommendations must now cover highly diverse populations, including those with chronic diseases and challenges to metabolic health. A systems perspective must be brought to bear when thinking about dietary requirements in the context of disease prevention and management. This systems orientation, explained Stover, requires a rethinking of biomarkers as integrative biomarkers that capture the interactions of all the nutrients within the system and all the other inherent biological factors, such as genetic variation. Furthermore, if aging is a risk factor for chronic disease, then investigators need to understand the biomarkers of aging and how nutrition or nutrient supply alters the aging trajectory toward health or disease.

Stover also noted that the committee for DRIs in chronic disease (NASEM, 2017a) established that any recommendation based on a chronic disease endpoint should have a moderate level of evidence using the GRADE (Grading of Recommendations Assessment, Development and Evaluation) system. He stated that this level of evidence sets a very high bar for the nutrition community, and that it exists for very few nutrient and chronic disease relationships.

Modifiers of Nutrient and Food Needs

The amount of nutrients required by an individual is determined by a number of physiological processes, including absorption, catabolism, excretion, metabolism, stability, transport, bio-activation, energetic state, and nutrient storage. Stover stated that all of these biological processes have modifiers and sensitizers, such as sex, pregnancy, lactation, age, the microbiome, pharmaceuticals, toxins, nutrient–nutrient interactions, genetics, food matrix, and epigenetics. All of these factors influence the physiological processes that determine nutrient needs and provide varia-

---

[5] This section summarizes information presented by Patrick Stover.

tions in requirements in the population. Disease can also be a major modifier of these processes.

Stover then illustrated current thinking about nutrient requirements for different populations (see Figure 1-2). For health and disease prevention, the DRIs capture the level of intake that is required to maintain whole body nutritional status, normal physiological function, or clinical outcomes in healthy people. Predictive biomarkers can be useful in determining nutrients that are needed currently and their effect on the risk, or onset, of chronic disease in the future. Recent estimates show that about half of the U.S. population suffers from, and is being treated for, a chronic disease (Ward et al., 2014). Based on this, Stover suggested that the DRIs may not be suitable for 50 percent of the U.S. population. Therefore, how should nutrient requirements in disease management be considered? For example, evidence may suggest that some of the comorbidities associated with a disease are due to the effect of that disease on nutritional status or nutritional function, which then increases susceptibility to other diseases. Diabetic neuropathy is a comorbidity that may be due to some sort of a nutrient deficiency related to the diabetes, Stover noted.

Tissue-specific nutritional status is also relevant. Sometimes, a disease is isolated to a single tissue and measuring and quantifying the nutritional needs of that diseased tissue in the absence of whole body indicators of the effect of a nutritional deficiency or nutritional excess can present a formidable challenge. Another issue in determining nutrient needs in a disease state is restoration of function that requires conditionally essential nutrients and tissue regeneration. A final consideration is that special nutritional requirements may optimize the number of stem cells avail-

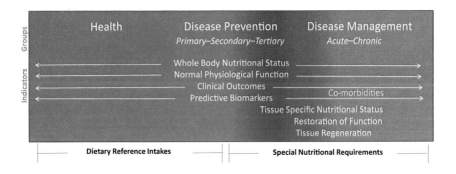

50% of the US adult population suffers from a chronic disease *Prev. Chronic. Dis.* 2014, 11, E62

FIGURE 1-2 Classifying and evaluating human nutrient needs.
SOURCE: As presented by Patrick Stover, April 2, 2018.

able, the quality of those stem cells, and their ability to restore an organ in terms of both the number of cells and their function.

Drugs, Nutrient Levels, and Biomarkers

Stover then noted that the effects of drugs on nutrient levels and their biomarkers need to be better understood and considered. Some examples are the effect of anti-hypertensives on folate levels; nonsteroidal anti-inflammatory drugs and aspirin on vitamin C and iron; hypoglycemics on vitamin B12, calcium, and vitamin D; and acid-suppressing drugs (proton pump inhibitors) on vitamin B12, vitamin C, iron, calcium, magnesium, and zinc.

Because fulfilling special nutritional needs is not equivalent to treating a primary disease, a relevant question is whether a nutrient intervention to respond to that special requirement may have a physiological or drug (i.e., an off-target) effect. Stover suggested that special nutritional needs act through evolutionarily derived physiological mechanisms to restore nutritional adequacy and physiological function, thereby managing a specific disease state, not through off-target effects. Niacin is an example of a nutrient that at pharmacological doses (i.e., 10 times the DRI[6]) improves lipid profiles, and it is not given because of a niacin deficiency. Therefore, niacin is not a special nutritional need but it is having an off-target effect that results in clinical improvement. Stover then set out the following considerations for proposed standards for special nutritional needs:

- A robust biological premise must be established. How and why are the nutritional needs different? What are the relevant biomarkers of these altered nutrient needs? Is it possible to use the same biomarkers for populations with a disease that are used with healthy populations?
- Efficacy must be addressed. Does the increased or decreased intake address disease-induced changes in nutrient needs? Does it affect nutritional status and/or nutrient function? Moreover, are these effects chronic or acute? Does the altered intake address any of the symptoms of the primary disease resulting from the nutritional deficiency and/or any comorbidities that are secondary to the primary disease, but that act through nutrition?
- Classification must be considered. What is the heterogeneity around nutritional requirements for any given disease or disease subtype?

---

[6] For DRI values, see http://nationalacademies.org/HMD/Activities/Nutrition/SummaryDRIs/DRI-Tables.aspx (accessed June 6, 2018).

All of the factors involved in disease-related etiology (e.g., inflammation in combination with genetic predisposition, autoimmunity, mitochondrial dysfunction, pharmaceuticals, and trauma) can influence physiological processes related to nutrition. Absorption, transport across the brain or nerve barriers, catabolism of nutrients, excretion of nutrients, altered metabolism, and altered distribution of nutrients among tissues can all be affected by a disease process and they affect human nutrition in terms of causing whole body deficiencies, tissue-specific deficiencies, and nutrient toxicities. These processes can also affect both the function and the status of biomarkers. Tissue-specific biomarkers of nutrient deficiency therefore become valuable ways to assess nutritional status. Predictive biomarkers that can reflect depleted nutrients and disease, progression of a disease, or progression of comorbidities related to that disease will all be needed, said Stover. An example of the complexities involved in factors that affect nutrient status and/or biomarkers of disease is acquired arginine deficiency syndrome, in which the enzyme arginase that degrades arginine is elevated. Infection, which results in tissue redistribution or excretion of nutrients such as iron, is another example.

Stover noted that a number of workshop speakers would address inborn errors of metabolism. These conditions, where nutrition compensates for functional deficits caused by genetics, may be a good model for considering nutrition in chronic disease. In the context of chronic disease, it may be possible to think about nutrition compensating for functional deficits caused by the disease.

The Cochrane PICO (Population, Intervention, Comparisons, Outcomes) approach provides a way to think about this, suggested Stover. Each of the PICO elements can be seen through the DRI or special nutritional needs lens (see Table 1-1).

Stover closed his presentation by noting that special nutritional requirements are an important area of research. When the American Society for Nutrition published its research agenda in 2013, it listed variability in responses to diet and medical management as two of its six research priority areas (ASN, 2013). The USA Interagency Committee on Human Nutrition Research included "How do we enhance our understanding of the role of nutrition in health promotion and disease prevention and treatment?" as the first question in its National Nutrition Research Roadmap 2016–2021 (ICHNR, 2016). Its second question was "How do we enhance our understanding of individual differences in nutritional status and variability in response to diet?"

TABLE 1-1 Comparison of Dietary Reference Intakes and Special Nutritional Needs

	DRI	Special Nutritional Needs
Population	Healthy populations Sex, age, pregnancy, lactation	Clinical populations Classifiable condition/disease
Intervention	Diet, dietary supplement	Needs may not be met by "diet" alone
Comparisons	Dose response	Dose response
Outcomes	Avoid nutrient deficiency, support physiological processes, and/or chronic disease prevention	Avoid disease-induced nutrient deficiency, support compromised physiological processes in disease and/or support tissue regeneration (dietary management of disease)

NOTE: DRI = Dietary Reference Intake.
SOURCE: As presented by Patrick Stover, April 2, 2018.

MODERATED PANEL DISCUSSION AND Q&A

In the discussion period following the Brannon and Stover presentations, participants addressed a variety of topics.

Characterizing Nutrients

The discussion highlighted the fact that the definition of a "nutrient" might be too narrow and panelists agree that using the broader term "nutrient and other food substance," as in the recent National Academies report on setting DRIs in chronic diseases (NASEM, 2017a) will be more helpful. Brannon envisioned a scenario in which a disease affects nutritional requirements or metabolism such that a bioactive food component might have an important role to play in managing those effects and it could influence nutrient distributions and other factors.

Virginia Stallings, Children's Hospital of Philadelphia, followed up by suggesting the related idea of a special dietary pattern that could influence the response of nutrients because of small, synergistic effects with bioactive food components.

Lessons from Research in Aging

Stover noted that investigators have shown that as people age, their epigenetic profiles decay. This decay results in more randomness in gene expression, which leads to functional decay in networks. Observational studies in aging populations show a correlation between the rate of decay of gene expression patterns or epigenetic landscape and the risk of chronic disease. Those whose epigenetic patterns decay more rapidly tend to have chronic diseases. Those who are able to retain earlier epigenetic signatures and gene expression profiles tend to age much more healthily. They have a lower biological age than their chronological age.

Stover continued that the role of nutrition in this environment is of considerable interest now. It is known that nutrition is essential in establishing embryonic epigenetic landscapes and work in fetal origins of disease suggests that what the mother eats affects what her child's epigenetic patterns will be. What is not known, he said, is whether nutrition can be used to reprogram stem cells so that they can repopulate an aging organ with a younger gene expression pattern that could lead to metrics with improved function.

Nutrients and Bioactive Food Components

Schneeman commented that, although fiber is not considered a nutrient, a DRI was established for a fiber AI based on disease risk reduction. She also thought that Stover's discussion of comorbidities, and the notion that they should be managed as part of the disease process, was a new and thought-provoking notion.

An attendee asked Brannon and Stover to comment on other functional substances derived from foods. These substances may not have DRIs but are known to have an effect on biomarkers. For example, whey protein is concentrated with transforming growth factor beta. Oral immunoglobulin formulations have been tested since 1972 for infectious neuropathy, inflammatory bowel disease, or even irritable bowel syndrome. Some probiotic formulations can help in managing a disease when they are combined.

Stover agreed that this question raises the intriguing issue of what a nutrient is and how to consider combinations of nutrients. It may not be possible to meet special nutritional requirements by diet alone. In that case, nutrient formulations must be carefully considered. Stover also noted that any consideration of the gut must include the microbiome. The connection between nutrition, gut health, and overall physiological health will not be fully understood until interactions with the microbiome are studied further.

Use of Biomarkers

On a participant's question related to the clinical implications of identifying and using biomarkers to improve nutritional management of disease states, Brannon responded that she is not aware of much work that links physical exams either by a physician or another health care practitioner or registered dietician nutritionist with special nutritional requirements. She suggested that continued work in this area will be part of the translational research that might be necessary to make progress. She agreed that integrating validated biomarkers or surrogate endpoints into clinical practice and diagnosis will be difficult.

Schneeman added that one of the critical needs in this area, and in nutrition generally, is the importance of validated biomarkers. For a regulatory process, she stated that it is particularly important that those biomarkers be validated as surrogate endpoints.

Levels of Evidence

The suggestion that at least a moderate grade of evidence is necessary for meaningful recommendations to inform clinical practice was discussed as an issue of particular importance in nutrition science because few large RCTs are available to inform this work, and the lack of convincing evidence is a concern. Brannon noted that, in her opinion, a need for moderate strength of evidence does not necessarily equate to conducting many RCTs but can be generated with congruent and consistent effects integrated across observational studies and RCTs. She added that one reason for recommending at least a moderate strength of evidence is that it is currently difficult to make policy on a lesser grade of evidence. Reflecting from his experience on the DRI and chronic disease committee, Stover added that the GRADE framework is the standard for evaluating medical data and making recommendations and, if the goal is to connect diet to health, a high standard of evidence is needed. Schneeman added that she serves on the World Health Organization (WHO) Nutrition Guidance Expert Advisory Group, which uses the GRADE system for evaluating evidence. She stated that WHO recognizes that grading the strength of the evidence is just one step in the process. Another critical element, she states, is the strength of the recommendation that can be made based on that evidence.

Translation to the Clinical Setting

Concerns were raised regarding the translation of special nutritional requirements to patients when a regulatory path currently does not exist to get that treatment to patients. Susan Berry, University of Minnesota, replied that this situation is very common in inherited metabolic diseases. Some in the field, she said, had misgivings about arginine becoming a drug because of the difficulties in setting up appropriate studies when the number of patients available is limited. This makes it very difficult to achieve an important but very high standard in nutritional requirements.

Schneeman added that in the current regulatory framework a statement that a compound will treat, cure, prevent, or manage disease makes that compound a drug or a medical device. To provide an alternative, the Orphan Drug Act created a category called medical foods. A 1996 *Federal Register* notice outlined FDA's thinking about what constituted a medical food and foods for special dietary uses, but the notice was eventually withdrawn and an approval process for medical foods does not currently exist. A manufacturer can declare a product to be a medical food, and if FDA does not agree with this determination, the agency may send a warning letter. Schneeman concluded by saying that if the concept of special nutrient requirements can be defined and is relevant to the criteria for medical foods, a framework is necessary that will allow the public to have confidence in the claims being made.

Personalized Nutrition

A question was raised about the use of technological innovation to meet individual needs of certain patients. Stover responded first, saying that disruptive technologies are likely to play an important role in the future. For example, the same paper microfluidic device that enables pregnancy tests is now being commercialized with chronic disease markers, nutritional status markers, and other markers. Individuals will have considerable personal data and will be able to get real-time readouts of their physiological status and disease status. Schneeman agreed, stating that advances in genetics and metabolomics will help to define smaller populations where unique or special nutrient needs can be examined and where personalized nutrition can be defined in a way that is meaningful to individuals.

REFERENCES

ASN (American Society for Nutrition). 2013. The American Society for Nutrition announces nutrition research needs and a statement on fiber: 6 nutrition research areas with greatest opportunity for health impact. *Nutrition Today* 48(5):189–190.

ICHNR (Interagency Committee on Human Nutrition Research). 2016. *National nutrition research roadmap 2016–2021: Advancing nutrition research to improve and sustain health.* Washington, DC: Interagency Committee on Human Nutrition Research.

NASEM (National Academies of Sciences, Engineering, and Medicine). 2017a. *Guiding principles for developing Dietary Reference Intakes based on chronic disease.* Washington, DC: The National Academies Press.

NASEM. 2017b. *Redesigning the process for establishing the* Dietary Guidelines for Americans. Washington, DC: The National Academies Press.

NASEM. 2018. *Nutrigenomics and the future of nutrition. Proceedings of a workshop—in brief.* Washington, DC: The National Academies Press.

Ward, B. W., J. S. Schiller, and R. A. Goodman. 2014. Multiple chronic conditions among US adults: A 2012 update. *Preventing Chronic Disease* 11:E62.

2

Addressing Nutrient Needs Due to Loss of Function in Genetic Diseases

Session 2 was moderated by Erin MacLeod, Director of Metabolic Nutrition at the Children's National Health System and a Planning Committee member. In the first presentation, Denise Ney, Professor of Nutritional Sciences and Affiliate Faculty Waisman Center at the University of Wisconsin–Madison, described the basis of nutritional needs in the genetic disorder phenylketonuria (PKU). The next speaker was Marni Falk, Executive Director of the Mitochondrial Medicine Frontier Program at the Children's Hospital of Philadelphia and Associate Professor in the Division of Human Genetics within the Department of Pediatrics at the University of Pennsylvania Perelman School of Medicine. Falk provided an overview of mitochondrial diseases and explained the nutritional challenges in managing them. The third presenter, Charles Venditti at the National Human Genome Research Institute, National Institutes of Health (NIH), discussed the contributions of nutrients in complex inborn errors of metabolism, using methylmalonic acidemia (MMA) as a case example. Rounding out the presentations was Sue Berry, Division Director for Genetics and Metabolism in the Department of Pediatrics at the University of Minnesota. Berry discussed some of the lessons learned from efforts at nutritional management of inborn errors of metabolism. The session concluded with a moderated panel discussion and questions and answers with workshop participants.

UNDERSTANDING THE BASIS OF NUTRITIONAL NEEDS IN PHENYLKETONURIA[1]

PKU is an autosomal recessive disease and its nutrient requirements are unique due to its genetic basis and inheritance, which affects requirements for phenylalanine (Phe) and tyrosine. It is caused by more than 800 mutations in the phenylalanine hydroxylase (PAH) gene. Ney opened her presentation by explaining that PKU is characterized by a deficiency in the conversion of Phe to tyrosine. It is managed with the low Phe diet. An individual with classical PKU often needs to restrict Phe intake to 300 to 500 milligrams per day, about 10 percent of typical intake. Tetrahydrobiopterin is an essential co-factor for PAH. In 2009, the U.S. Food and Drug Administration (FDA) approved a drug called Kuvan, which provides a synthetic form of the tetrahydrobiopterin co-factor. Up to 20 to 50 percent of individuals with PKU, who have some residual PAH activity, respond to this co-factor supplementation with a decrease in plasma Phe, which allows them to increase their dietary Phe intake.

Evidence suggests both causality and an intake–response relationship with respect to the toxicity of Phe in PKU. Phe intake that exceeds anabolic needs increases Phe concentrations in blood and brain, resulting in profound cognitive impairment if PKU is not treated with a low Phe diet started shortly after birth. Maternal PKU results in impaired fetal development and congenital anomalies if the mother does not strictly control her blood Phe levels during pregnancy. The biomarker that is used clinically is blood Phe concentration, a surrogate for brain Phe concentration.

A PKU scientific review conference held by NIH used a data analysis from the Agency for Healthcare Research and Quality to conclude that moderate evidence exists for a threshold effect that a blood Phe level of 400 micromolar or greater is associated with IQs less than 85 (Lindegren et al., 2012). The current recommendation in the United States is lifelong treatment of PKU, with a goal of maintaining blood Phe in the range of 120 to 360 micromolar.

Low Phe Diet

Ney described that the low Phe diet for PKU is adhered to fairly well in early childhood, when rapid development occurs. However, lifelong compliance is very challenging. The diet has the following components:

---

[1] This section summarizes information presented by Denise Ney.

- Elimination of all high-protein foods. This means no animal foods or high-protein vegetable foods, such as seeds, nuts, and legumes.
- Protein substitution and micronutrient supplementation with medical foods. In 1958, the first low-Phe formula for PKU, Lofenalac, was introduced in the United States. Lofenalac is formulated from a casein hydrolysate. This was followed in 1972 by formulations comprising mixtures of amino acids leaving out Phe, and these were designated as medical foods in 1988. A second type of medical food, introduced in 2010, uses the peptide, glycomacropeptide (GMP), a 64-amino acid glycophosphopeptide. GMP is found in milk within the K-casein micelle and contains no Phe in its pure form.

The Genetic Metabolic Dietitians International Organization has developed dietary recommendations for PKU (Singh et al., 2016). The organization recommends a 20 to 50 percent higher protein intake when amino acid medical foods provide the primary source of protein, based on the body's rapid absorption and oxidation of amino acids, resulting in reduced protein synthesis. Ney noted that improved growth in children with PKU who are fed protein at levels above the Recommended Dietary Allowance[2] has been documented. This principle is relevant to gastrointestinal (GI) conditions where amino acid and peptide formulations are used.

Phe Tolerance or Minimum Phe Requirement

For an individual with classical PKU (i.e., a virtual absence of activity in the PAH gene), the Phe tolerance, or minimum Phe requirement, is the amount of Phe needed for protein synthesis to support growth and maintenance. Several studies have established the Phe requirements for infants from birth to 3 months. The first Collaborative Study, based on food records and multiple Phe determinations for blood, showed the requirements were 55 to 62 mg Phe/kg/d (Acosta et al., 1977). These findings paralleled those of Fomon and Filer, which showed 42 to 61 mg/Phe/kg/d are required to support the growth of healthy infants (Fomon and Filer, 1967). After 3 months of age, minimum Phe requirements are lower for PKU compared to the Dietary Reference Intakes (DRIs).[3]

In contrast, nutrient requirements for individuals older than 4 years with PKU are poorly determined. Several approaches are used to establish Phe tolerance for adults with classical PKU. Using intensive dietary

---

[2] For DRI values, see http://nationalacademies.org/HMD/Activities/Nutrition/Summary DRIs/DRI-Tables.aspx (accessed June 6, 2018).

[3] For DRI values, see http://nationalacademies.org/HMD/Activities/Nutrition/Summary DRIs/DRI-Tables.aspx (accessed June 6, 2018).

counseling, along with food records and blood Phe determinations over a period of several months, Phe tolerance can be increased from about 5 to about 8.5 milligrams per kilogram per day (MacLeod et al., 2009), about one-third the most current amino acid requirements of 25 milligrams of a combination of Phe and tyrosine (FAO/WHO/UNU Expert Consultation, 2007). Observations from clinical trials suggest that this low level of Phe intake can be difficult to maintain by adult individuals.

Tyrosine Requirements in Phenylketonuria

Tyrosine requirements in PKU are poorly understood. As the primary substrate for the synthesis of the catecholamine neurotransmitters, the low levels of tyrosine often seen in PKU patients is a concern. The response is to supplement their diet with tyrosine. Ney's research has shown that the prebiotic GMP improves the bioavailability of tyrosine in PKU.

Ney went on to explain that despite almost 50 percent lower intake of tyrosine with GMP compared to amino acid medical foods, fasting plasma tyrosine levels are not different and within the normal range. These findings were reinforced by a 13-month study from Portugal that demonstrated increased mean blood tyrosine levels in study participants with PKU using daily servings of GMP medical foods (Pinto et al., 2017).

A metabolomics analysis revealed that the tyrosine is converted by the gut bacteria to potentially harmful compounds, in this case, tyramine and phenol sulfate, which are associated with headaches and renal toxicity, respectively (Ney et al., 2017). The use of pre- and probiotic supplements to decrease the gut synthesis of these renal toxins is a common element of disease management in people with chronic renal disease.

Phenylketonuria and Conditionally Essential Nutrients

PKU is likely associated with conditionally essential nutrients. People with PKU have low cholesterol levels, possibly as a result of lower cholesterol biosynthesis due to changes in metabolism associated with high blood levels of Phe. Inflammation and oxidative stress observed in PKU likely affect nutrient requirements. Lastly, low levels of several nutrients are observed in PKU, especially in children with the condition.

In addition, low bone mineral density and increased risk of fractures have emerged as complications of treated PKU, which may be associated with the high dietary acid load in amino acid medical foods. Studies in healthy individuals demonstrate that chronic ingestion of a high dietary acid load is bad for bone, which provides a very large bicarbonate reservoir and assists the kidneys in maintaining systemic pH homeostasis. This concept is especially important with age-related declines in kidney function.

Ney's research group has confirmed these observations in a pilot cross-over trial of eight individuals with PKU where they determined that renal net acid excretion in 24-hour urine samples was threefold higher with ingestion of amino acid compared to GMP medical foods (Stroup et al., 2017). In addition, calcium excretion was significantly increased outside of the normal range compared to GMP with similar intake of calcium and bone-related nutrients.

Ney concluded her presentation with the following summary points:

- Nutrient requirements for protein, Phe, and tyrosine are unique in PKU.
- The principles of nutritional management of PKU have relevance to chronic disease, in particular, increased protein requirements with amino acid–based diets, as are often required in GI disorders.
- More needs to be learned about how the unique nutritional management approaches in conditions like PKU affect the gut microbiota, in particular, nutrient bioavailability, the synthesis of both beneficial metabolites, such as short-chain fatty acids, and also potentially harmful metabolites.
- The concept of conditionally essential nutrients in PKU, with altered metabolism and inflammation or oxidative stress, dietary acid load, and bone health, also has relevance for chronic conditions.
- Even though PKU is a mono-genetic disorder, it still has tremendous genetic diversity, which suggests substantial variation in nutrient requirements within the PKU population.

NUTRITIONAL INADEQUACIES IN MITOCHONDRIAL-ASSOCIATED METABOLIC DISORDERS[4]

Mitochondria are sub-cellular cytoplasmic organelles that arose about 2 billion years ago from purple sulfur cyanobacteria. They play a major role in nearly every metabolic pathway involved in oxidation of nutrients to permit cell growth and function. In addition to their major function as the energy "powerhouse" of the cell, Falk explained that mitochondria have central roles in many other essential activities, including calcium homeostasis and apoptosis.

Mitochondrial Disease

Falk stated that due to their broad range of functions, mitochondrial malfunction can cause symptoms in any organ at any age by any mode

---

[4] This section summarizes information presented by Marni Falk.

of inheritance. This multiplicity of effects created a long-standing skepticism about mitochondrial disease, which is gradually disappearing. Many people have tried to identify a universal biomarker for mitochondrial disease, but unfortunately, no single biomarker exists because of the many different genes that can be involved in causing mitochondrial diseases.

Gene mutations that cause primary mitochondrial disease may occur both in the deoxyribonucleic acid (DNA) within the mitochondrion itself and in nuclear DNA. More than 20 novel gene disorders that are recognized to cause mitochondrial disease have been identified each year for the past decade. Although each individual gene cause is fairly uncommon, mitochondrial disease as a whole is the most common inborn error of metabolism, affecting at least 1 in 4,300 people across all ages.

Although it has been known since the 1950s that mitochondrial disease involves dysfunction in the energy-generating pathway that occurs within mitochondria, it is now recognized that mitochondrial disease may involve many additional processes and pathways occurring within these organelles (see Figure 2-1).

Clinical Features of Mitochondrial Disease

In describing mitochondrial disease, Falk noted that a wide range of organs may be affected, although most patients do have some form of neurologic and/or muscle involvement. Indeed, the disease can affect any one of the four nervous systems, that is, the central, peripheral, autonomic, and GI nervous systems. In addition to neurologic problems, whose onset may occur at any age and range from headaches and balance problems to Parkinson's or developmental regression, eye problems such as drooping eyelid, eye muscle movement problems, and vision loss from retinal and/or optic nerve dysfunction are very common. Heart muscle or rhythm problems either as the sole feature or as part of a progressive multi-system array of problems that develop over time can also occur. Other common problems include fatigue, exercise intolerance, muscle weakness, developmental delay, sensorineural hearing loss, GI dysmotility, liver problems, kidney problems, bone marrow insufficiency, infertility, acute metabolic instability, and a host of endocrine problems.

Therapies for Mitochondrial Disease

No proven effective therapies or cures for mitochondrial disease are available, mostly because it consists of so many individually rare, highly heterogeneous disorders. Exercise, both aerobic and isotonic, has been shown for about a decade to have therapeutic value, but clarity on an optimal diet is lacking. So-called mitochondrial supplement cocktails

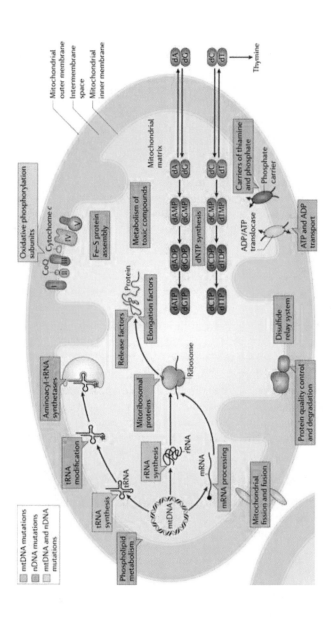

FIGURE 2-1 Mitochondrial disease: Molecular pathways affected by genetic disorders.

NOTE: ADP = adenosine diphosphate; ATP = adenosine triphosphate; DNA = deoxyribonucleic acid; Fe = iron; mRNA = messenger RNA; mtDNA = mitochondrial DNA; nDNA = nuclear DNA; rRNA = ribosomal RNA; S = sulfur; tRNA = transfer RNA.

SOURCES: As presented by Marni Falk, April 2, 2018; Gorman et al., 2016. Reprinted by permission from Springer Nature. *Nature Reviews Disease Primers*. Mitochondrial diseases, Gorman, G. S., P. F. Chinnery, S. DiMauro, M. Hirano, Y. Koga, R. McFarland, A. Suomalainen, D. R. Thorburn, M. Zeviani, and D. M. Turnbull, Copyright 2016. https://www.nature.com/nrdp (accessed June 14, 2018).

have been empirically used for some time based on the supposition they beneficially affect mitochondrial enzymes and cellular stress. These one-size-fits-all cocktails have great variability in their composition and clinical use, Falk stated. They commonly include

- supplements to increase free coenzyme Q pool (carnitine, pantothenate);
- enzyme co-factors (vitamins B1 or B2);
- metabolite therapies (arginine, folinic acid, creatine);
- enzyme activators (dicholoroacetate); and
- antioxidants (vitamins C or E, lipoic acid, coenzyme Q).

For the past decade, amino acid therapies have focused on arginine and citrulline. In some patients with mitochondrial disease, such as the common mitochondrial DNA syndrome called MELAS (mitochondrial encephalopathy, lactic acidosis, and stroke-like episodes), acute stroke-like episodes have been shown to be mitigated with intravenous arginine. An expert consensus panel (Parikh et al., 2015) considered its use and determined that overall, it is well tolerated when administered at the proper doses and the patient is monitored for potential occurrence of low blood pressure and low blood sugar. A clinical trial is now under way to compare intravenous arginine and citrulline for treatment of acute stroke-like episodes in MELAS patients. Enteral arginine or citrulline is also commonly used as a prophylactic agent for acute metabolic stroke occurring in mitochondrial disease.

Clinical trials are now emerging, but as yet no universal clinical trial design, outcome measure, or biomarker has been established. Most of these trials have pursued antioxidant therapies for clinical syndromes, but without clear positive results. Newer agents are now under study in a range of clinical syndromes with a growing variety of therapeutic agents.

Nutritional Guidance in Mitochondrial Disease

To improve nutrition, many patients with mitochondrial disease may require a gastrostomy tube or parental nutrition, which is often associated with swallowing disorders, abnormal gut motility, and other GI complications. It is also known that essential micronutrient deficiencies may occur, including those of vitamin B12, vitamin D, folate, zinc, and others. Falk noted that multivitamin supplements safely alleviate some of these potential deficiencies, and that lutein is used in some cases if there is ophthalmologic involvement of the optic nerve or retina. However, she stated that very limited guidance is available to guide most aspects of nutrition in mitochondrial disease. No scientific data are available to support guidance of optimal feeding intervals or specific macronutrient profiles involving the desired dietary ratio of proteins, carbohydrates, or fat. Although this issue has generated considerable discussion, current expert consensus recommendations do not include any clarity on the macronutrient profile. Current guidance suggests that energy, protein, and micronutrient intake should be evaluated and relative under-nutrition should be assessed in light of issues such as altered energy expenditures, abnormal intake, and absorption.

Because the glycolytic rate is typically increased in mitochondrial disease, high-carbohydrate diets may be beneficial. Furthermore, patients with acute metabolic stressors that may cause neurodevelopmental regression with decompensation, such as a fever or an infection, are often given glucose-containing fluids to prevent catabolism. Concerns have arisen about acute glucose infusion precipitating a metabolic crisis due to the increased nicotinamide adenine dinucleotide + hydrogen (NADH) to nicotinamide adenine dinucleotide (NAD) ratio that occurs in mitochondrial disease. A study being performed by Shana McCormack at the Children's Hospital of Philadelphia's Mitochondrial Medicine Frontier Program suggests that the type of carbohydrate may matter, as low-glycemic carbohydrates may offer a means to improve health outcomes and cognition in adult patients with genetically confirmed mitochondrial disease. Another concern is that diabetes mellitus is common in some patients. Falk concluded that even though glucose or low-glycemic carbohydrates might be possible therapies, much still needs to be learned about their optimization for acute and chronic care of patients with mitochondrial disease. The ketogenic diet (very high fat and very low carbohydrate) has been reported as a possible therapeutic approach for mitochondrial disease, particularly in patients with intractable epilepsy. By increasing ketones, succinate, and the starvation response, mitochondria biogenesis is increased and glutathione metabolism is enhanced. However, its clinical use is controversial due to inconclusive results from animal model studies. A major complicating factor is that the ketogenic diet is often not tolerated in patients because they metabolize fat poorly. Concerns also exist about the long-term health risks of the ketogenic diet. The modified Atkins diet, which involves a less extreme but still relatively high-fat and low-carbohydrate diet, has also been tried. A recent Finnish trial showed that although ten healthy adult control subjects had no problem completing a 4-week trial, all five mitochondrial myopathy adult subjects stopped the diet early due to severe muscle pain and burning as well as headaches and increased fatigue (Ahola et al., 2016). The explanation for this adverse response, stated Falk, was the impaired ability of mitochondrial myopathy study participants' muscle fibers to burn fat aerobically in mitochondria, as they have upregulated activity of their anaerobic glycolysis pathway to use sugar directly to generate energy.

Other nutritional recommendations include general common sense, such as having well-balanced diets with a range of fruits and vegetables, taking a multivitamin, avoiding fasting, and encouraging frequent small meals. In addition, good fluid intake is recommended, with increased fluid given when needed for heat, activity, or metabolic stress occurs.

Novel Treatment Strategies

Novel treatment strategies being considered to treat mitochondrial disease include genetic correction strategies as well as small molecular approaches, metabolic manipulation, and diet and exercise to treat the secondary cell consequences of the disease. Thinking about the mitochondrial respiratory chain as a "black box" factory that generates certain products, such as free radicals, adenosine triphosphate (ATP), nucleic acids, and nicotinamide dinucleotides, investigators are now looking at therapies that may not target the mitochondrial function proximally but, rather, focus on alleviating the resulting downstream deficiencies and broader cellular effects. The approach might involve activating certain signaling networks and biological processes, such as the mechanistic target of rapamycin complex 1 (mTORC1)-mediated control of cytosolic translation and autophagy. These processes are often dysregulated in mitochondrial disease, leading to a state of increased cellular stress. Falk showed a schematic illustrating this approach (see Figure 2-2).

Falk's research laboratory group has tested more than three dozen antioxidants, metabolic modifiers, and signaling modifiers in a well-validated *Caenorhabditis elegans* (*C. elegans*) worm model of genetic-based primary mitochondrial disease. In each of these three treatment classes, some key therapies significantly restored the animals' short lifespan. For example, lead signaling modifiers were nicotinic acid and probucol, and glucose was an effective metabolic therapy, as were the antioxidants N-acetylcysteine and vitamin E. The beneficial effects of each of these molecules when administered individually has been validated in vertebrate zebrafish animal models of primary mitochondrial disease.

Indeed, Falk's group and many investigators around the world are evaluating different molecules and approaches (e.g., nutritional variation, drugs, and genetic therapies) in a wide variety of model animals and human cell types, testing their effects on biochemical as well as clinically relevant outcomes, such as survival, function, and feeling. Translational pre-clinical studies may also allow improved understanding of biomarkers for different molecular subtypes of mitochondrial disease. The results from this pre-clinical work have the potential to be used to devise a personalized

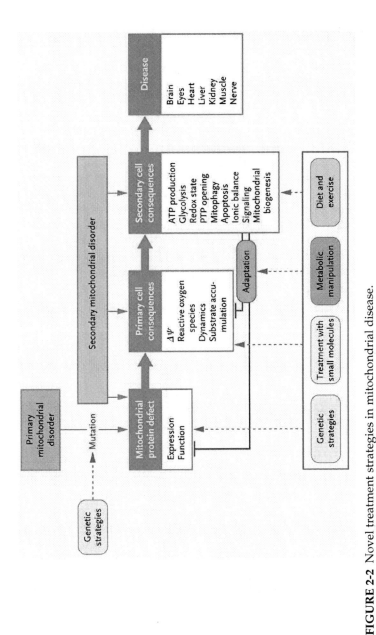

FIGURE 2-2 Novel treatment strategies in mitochondrial disease.

NOTE: ATP = adenosine triphosphate; PTP = permeability transition pore.

SOURCES: As presented by Marni Falk, April 2, 2018; Koopman et al., 2012. From the *New England Journal of Medicine.* Koopman, W. J., P. H. Willems, and J. A. Smeitink. Monogenic mitochondrial disorders. Volume 366, page 1139. Copyright 2012. Massachusetts Medical Society. Reprinted with permission from Massachusetts Medical Society.

trial that objectively tests the therapy in a given patient or for a disease type. In Falk's own research, some combined therapy combinations, or cocktails, appear to have synergistic effects.

Falk concluded with the following major summary points that reflect her own current thinking about therapeutic approaches to managing patients with mitochondrial disease:

- Some classical mitochondrial cocktail therapies do have objective therapeutic value in primary mitochondrial disease. However, their true value needs to be recognized as drugs intended to restore a state of health in genetically programmed mitochondrial diseases, rather than as unregulated dietary supplements that are intended for health optimization in the general, healthy population. Synergies between therapy components may be possible, if the proper doses, combinations, and unique mechanisms to treat different aspects of the disease pathophysiology can be identified.
- It is ideal to model therapies, when possible, in different mitochondrial disease subtypes before trying them empirically in clinic or prioritizing any one treatment randomly for further evaluation in a clinical treatment trial of mitochondrial disease patients. A promising diet to consider evaluating in primary mitochondrial disease patients may be one that is low glycemic and high carbohydrate rather than one that is high fat.
- It will be essential to evaluate the multiple potential clinical effects of dietary and nutrient therapies, to identify which aspects of these complex multi-systemic diseases respond and which clinical improvements are most valued by patients.

CONTRIBUTION OF NUTRIENTS IN COMPLEX INBORN ERRORS OF METABOLISM: THE CASE OF METHYLMALONIC ACIDEMIA[5]

MMA is a disorder of essential amino acid and odd chain fatty acid metabolism in humans. In essence, Venditti explained, four of the amino acids that are metabolized by the Krebs cycle—methionine, isoleucine, threonine, and valine, which are called propiogenic amino acids—cannot be oxidized because they lack their co-factor ado-cbl and instead they produce toxic acids in the body, such as methylmalonic acid. In MMA, the pathway to form ado-cbl from hydroxylcobalamin in the diet is aberrant. In the classical forms of MMA, patients have as much as 10,000 times the upper limit of normal methylmalonic acid in a healthy individual. MMA is the extreme end of a spectrum of metabolic perturbations related to

---

[5] This section summarizes information presented by Charles Venditti.

vitamin B12 metabolism. MMA patients have a variety of symptoms and affected organs. All the patients eventually develop chronic renal failure and most patients have poor growth and obesity. The most worrisome aspect of MMA is that patients have a phenomenon of metabolic instability in which they can decompensate and die rapidly when they are subjected to stress, infection, or dietary indiscretion.

The definitive therapy for MMA, which is not yet available, is a gene or cell therapy that gives back the dysfunctional enzyme in every cell. The only real treatment that is offered to children with classical isolated MMA is an elective liver transplant procedure. A combined liver and kidney transplant is also done. Medical nutritional management with metabolites derived from valine, isoleucine, and odd chain fatty acids is used globally. Patients can also be given antibiotics to sterilize their GI tract to reduce the amount of propionate and in turn methylmalonic acid. An additional management option is to try to detoxify and relieve coenzyme A accretion by giving high doses of carnitine. Another approach, although its effectiveness is unknown, is to try to make the Krebs cycle work more efficiently by giving citrate. Mitochondrial target therapies can also be used in an effort to mitigate the electron transport chain effects.

Medical Nutrition Therapy to Treat Methylmalonic Acidemia

As mentioned, a frequent diet for MMA patients is a relatively low protein diet to restrict the propiogenic precursors, the amino acids valine, isoleucine, methionine, or threonine, and a medical food also without those amino acids (Manoli et al., 2016a,b). Venditti described a few studies that illustrated his concerns with management of these patients with medical foods that have not been designed appropriately. He explained an NIH study that followed a cohort of about 200 patients with various forms of MMA (www.ClinicalTrials.gov: NCT00078078) to understand patterns in the disease based on the subjects' clinical phenotypes. Vendetti then presented data with results from this patient cohort, showing patient age and protein or equivalent, in grams per patient per day (see Figure 2-3).

The data show that some patients who were not hypermetabolic, and who should have been protein restricted, were in fact tolerating intakes far beyond the DRI[6] (many of them at 200 percent of the DRI; see Figure 2-3). Venditti wondered whether the fact that these patients did not grow could be related to their diet, which had led to an imbalance in the metabolism of branched chain amino acids. As it turned out, the patients were prescribed medical foods formulas that contained four to

---

[6] For DRI values, see http://nationalacademies.org/HMD/Activities/Nutrition/Summary DRIs/DRI-Tables.aspx (accessed June 6, 2018).

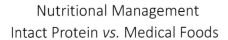

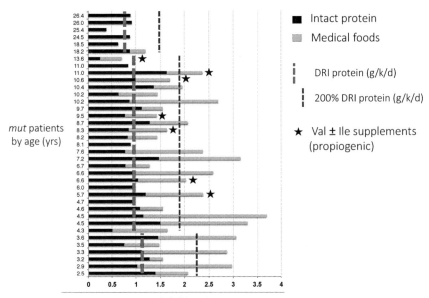

Protein or equivalent (g/k/d) - of **ACTUAL** weight!

FIGURE 2-3 Daily protein intake (grams/kilogram/day) by patients with methylmalonic acidemia (MMA) *mut* subtype sorted by age.

NOTES: The patients were given either an intact protein (black lines) or medical foods (gray lines). The DRI reference value and 200 percent of the reference value are provided as reference. Bars with a star * denote individuals who were given valine and isoleucine (propiogenic amino acids) as a supplement due to persistently low plasma amino acid concentration. DRI = Dietary Reference Intake; ile = isoleucine; val = valine.

SOURCES: As presented by Charles Venditti, April 2, 2018; Manoli et al., 2016a. Reprinted by permission from Springer Nature. *Genetics in Medicine*. A critical reappraisal of dietary practices in methylmalonic acidemia raises concerns about the safety of medical foods. Part 1: Isolated methylmalonic acidemias. Manoli, I., J. G. Myles, J. L. Sloan, O. A. Shchelochkov, and C. P. Venditti. Copyright 2015.

five times the DRI for leucine and zero isoleucine and valine (to prevent them from being propiogenic). However, Venditti's analysis showed that the branched chain amino acid ratios in these patients were altered, probably because of the intake of medical foods. A further correlative analysis showed an inverse relationship between the level of medical foods intake and the levels of valine and isoleucine in these patients.

Furthermore, the more medical foods a patient took, the more aberrant the branch amino acids ratio became and the poorer the growth was.

A possible explanation is that the unbalanced leucine load in these patients likely promoted a decrease in isoleucine and valine. When the patient's blood was too low in isoleucine and valine levels, an erroneous decision was made to supplement with isoleucine and valine. Valine and isoleucine are toxic precursors of methylmalonic acid. Venditti's research group and other centers have been able to correct the branched chain amino acids deficiency syndromes in MMA patients by lowering the medical foods and lowering amino acid intake (Manoli et al., 2016a,b).

Venditti concluded his presentation with the following summary points:

- Medical foods are specially designed to treat patients with inborn errors of metabolism or other medical conditions, but too much can produce an iatrogenic toxicity syndrome in MMA.
- Reformulation of some of the medical foods and testing for effects on oxidation should be conducted to determine whether amounts given are perturbing amino acid levels.
- Research and other proof of concept studies are indicated for medical foods.

LESSONS LEARNED: WHAT IS KNOWN ABOUT NUTRITION MANAGEMENT FOR INBORN ERRORS OF METABOLISM[7]

As discussed in earlier presentations, inborn errors of metabolism are a large class of genetic disorders. They are typically single-gene abnormalities that are primarily nuclear and very few are maternally inherited. Essentially, the errors are failures to synthesize a product or a failure in catabolism, primarily due to single enzymes in those pathways, and are sometimes associated with enzyme co-factors, such as those in MMA. Elaborating, Berry explained that the primary focus of clinical attention is on the consequences of these errors in metabolism. These can be of several types, including

- decreases in product, such as in PKU;
- increases in precursors; this is true for PKU and even more so in MMA, where the tremendous increases in precursors can have toxic effects; and
- shunts to alternative pathways, as in orotic acid in urea cycle disorders; in some cases, these shunts can be used diagnostically.

---

[7] This section summarizes information presented by Sue Berry.

Categories of Metabolic Diseases Where Nutrition Influences Care

Barry noted that metabolic diseases can also be grouped in terms of nutritional impact, including

- disorders of protein metabolism, such as PKU and MMA;
- disorders of carbohydrate metabolism, such as galactosemia;
- disorders of failure to generate glucose, such as glycogen storage diseases;
- fatty acid oxidation disorders, such as those involving failure to generate ketones; and
- mitochondrial disorders.

Treatment generally involves restricting or supplementing. Adequate calorie intake also needs to be ensured and this often involves providing substantial amounts of glucose. Monitoring nutrient adequacy is another key aspect of managing patients with these disorders. For example, clinicians must make sure protein is sufficient, but not excessive, in the protein disorders. Patients need to have enough essential fatty acids and may become very sick if fats are overly restricted in fatty acid oxidation disorders. Co-factor supplementation is another very important consideration in some cases. Scavenger therapies to get rid of undesired compounds have been used but need to be used carefully. Berry then suggested two additional strategies: monitoring toxic metabolites (i.e., keeping track of whether treatment is having the desired effect) and paying attention to biomarkers. Finally, clinicians must keep in mind that acute events inevitably occur, with various metabolic results.

Managing Inborn Errors of Metabolism

Reflecting on the preceding presentations in Session 2, Berry then described some of the issues that make the management of inborn errors of metabolism such a complex balancing act.

Phenylketonuria

In PKU, preventing the neurotoxic accumulation of Phe is the key management strategy. Some treatments, such as valine, isoleucine, and leucine, have been used to interfere with the transport of the amino acid Phe into the brain. In the early days of treating PKU, children died because all Phe was restricted; tyrosine then became a relative essential amino acid in that setting because Phe was restricted. This also proved that co-factors can be effective in some cases. Tetrahydrobiopterin, used in treating PKU, is an example of how a co-factor can have a tremendous impact on care.

Berry added that the spectrum of the phenotype is very important in thinking about PKU as a paradigm disease. For example, the most severely affected patients with PKU will have a very limited tolerance of protein. In contrast, patients who have slightly milder mutations can be more generous in their protein consumption. This issue also highlights concerns about conditional essentially nutrients, especially in catabolic states. As PKU treatments have improved, clinicians have developed a better understanding of micronutrients that they previously did not consider. For example, initial issues encountered in selenium, zinc, and other deficiencies have now been resolved.

Mitochondrial Disorders

Both primary and secondary mitochondrial impacts are important in thinking about diet-related treatment approaches. No defined optimal diet exists for mitochondrial-associated disorders and few trials have examined this issue. The primary target for mitochondrial diseases is to maximize appropriate dietary components, including energy and micronutrients; avoid fasting and dehydration; and consider antioxidants. A limited number of mitochondrial disorders have a specific or diet co-factor need and in those cases, supplying these co-factors is very important.

Because the compounds used as primary intervention for mitochondrial diseases are currently being thought of more as treatments than as supplements, issues of access and availability need to be addressed.

Methylmalonic Acidemia

Berry stated that Venditti provided an excellent review of the importance of targeting medical foods to a disease so they do not result in amino acid imbalances. She noted that the lack of sufficiently large cohorts and the lack of financial resources to study these issues are difficult problems to resolve. In MMA, poor growth and obesity outcomes are related to the failure to understand the broad spectrum of nutritional needs in these children.

Comparing Inborn Errors of Metabolism and Normal Nutritional Needs

Berry reflected on clinicians' responsibility to strike a balance in terms of nutrient needs in inherited metabolic diseases because the nutrient deficits are based on the individual disorder (e.g., tyrosine in PKU). The clinician's job is to manage patients so they achieve intakes that are very close to the required minimum; much still needs to be learned about how to strike this balance optimally. The use of artificial diets runs the risk of limiting micronutrients. Berry also reflected on the importance of the delivery method. For example, in the case of delivering amino acids, protein, or nitrogen equivalent, total parenteral nutrition is not an optimal way to give whole protein to patients.

Berry then described several key challenges in treating inborn errors of metabolism: (1) cost and access; (2) effects of treatments on the microbiome (the Urea Cycle Disease Consortium has a large project devoted to thinking about gut microbiome and its impact in the urea cycle disorder); (3) the need for medical foods to be optimally constituted and disorder-specific; and (4) the fact that nutritional needs change throughout the patient's lifespan.

In terms of what is next in nutrition care for inborn errors of metabolism, she provided the following perspective:

- Huge gaps in information and knowledge still exist because of a dearth of longitudinal follow-up to determine natural history in inherited metabolic diseases, and a lack of clinical trials.
- Medical foods and supplements are not covered by insurance. This represents a tremendous burden on families.
- Research funding is desperately needed to determine whether some of these observations are generalizable to other rare disorders and micronutrient needs.

MODERATED PANEL DISCUSSION AND Q&A

In the discussion period following these presentations, participants addressed a variety of topics.

Efficacy of Alternative Medicine

The presenters were asked about the efficacy of traditional Chinese medicines for treating inherited metabolic disorders. Falk said that one of the limiting factors in studying these diseases is creating models and having well-defined and well-phenotyped patients. Advances in animal models are allowing researchers to systematically test potential compounds in high-throughput drug screens. In her opinion, over the next few years, systematic tests are needed of different compounds, different natural food products, and drugs to isolate the components that might have effects. Merely thinking about food or Eastern or Western medicine is not as helpful as thinking about the components, she said, and whether a component is really therapeutically effective.

Nutrients, Drugs, and the Regulatory Process

Several participants and panelists discussed the complexities of testing products that address distinctive nutritional requirements and how that intersects with the current regulatory structure for approving drugs for treatment. For example, no structure or patent protection exists to allow companies to develop drugs made from natural molecules. The current structure requires companies to file Investigational New Drug applications with FDA, which represents a risk for the companies.

Falk said it is a real worry that medical foods, which patients rely on to maintain their lives and improve their health, are not being regulated properly and resulting in unnecessary deaths on occasion. Collaboration is needed by all to create a better framework that results in well-regulated products that do not impose an undue financial burden on families. Falk said she thought it is important to change current thinking about how products are approved and how to define the populations for whom treatments are developed. For example, carnitine is an essential treatment in fatty acid oxidation diseases, but it is shown to lead to coronary artery disease in people in the general population who take it over time. The clinical and research communities need to better define the target populations for therapies, she said. Therapies need to be developed and regulated properly and made available to patients. Berry and Venditti both agreed with a participant's comment about the value of medical foods and the need for research to improve them.

REFERENCES

Acosta, P. B., E. Wenz, and M. Williamson. 1977. Nutrient intake of treated infants with phenylketonuria. *American Journal of Clinical Nutrition* 30(2):198–208.

Ahola, S., M. Auranen, P. Isohanni, S. Niemisalo, N. Urho, J. Buzkova, V. Velagapudi, N. Lundbom, A. Hakkarainen, T. Muurinen, P. Piirila, K. H. Pietilainen, and A. Suomalainen. 2016. Modified Atkins diet induces subacute selective ragged-red-fiber lysis in mitochondrial myopathy patients. *EMBO Molecular Medicine* 8(11):1234–1247.

FAO/WHO/UNU (Food and Agriculture Organization of the United Nations/World Health Organization/United Nations University) Expert Consultation. 2007. *Protein and amino acid requirements in human nutrition. Report of a joint FAO/WHO/UNU expert consultation.* Geneva, Switzerland: World Health Organization. http://www.who.int/iris/handle/10665/43411 (accessed May 10, 2018).

Fomon, S. J., and L. J. Filer. 1967. Amino acid requirements for normal growth. In *Amino acid metabolism and genetic variation,* edited by W. L. Nyhan. New York: McGraw-Hill.

Gorman, G. S., P. F. Chinnery, S. DiMauro, M. Hirano, Y. Koga, R. McFarland, A. Suomalainen, D. R. Thorburn, M. Zeviani, and D. M. Turnbull. 2016. Mitochondrial diseases. *Nature Reviews Disease Primers* 2:16080.

Koopman, W. J., P. H. Willems, and J. A. Smeitink. 2012. Monogenic mitochondrial disorders. *New England Journal of Medicine* 366(12):1132–1141.

Lindegren, M. L., S. Krishnaswami, C. Fonnesbeck, T. Reimschisel, J. Fisher, K. Jackson, T. Shields, N. A. Sathe, and M. L. McPheeters. 2012. *Adjuvant treatment for phenylketonuria (PKU). Comparative Effectiveness Reviews*, No. 56. Rockville, MD: Agency for Healthcare Research and Quality.

MacLeod, E. L., S. T. Gleason, S. C. van Calcar, and D. M. Ney. 2009. Reassessment of phenylalanine tolerance in adults with phenylketonuria is needed as body mass changes. *Molecular Genetics and Metabolism* 98(4):331–337.

Manoli, I., J. G. Myles, J. L. Sloan, O. A. Shchelochkov, and C. P. Venditti. 2016a. A critical reappraisal of dietary practices in methylmalonic acidemia raises concerns about the safety of medical foods. Part 1: Isolated methylmalonic acidemias. *Genetics in Medicine* 18(4):386–395.

Manoli, I., J. G. Myles, J. L. Sloan, N. Carrillo-Carrasco, E. Morava, K. A. Strauss, H. Morton, and C. P. Venditti. 2016b. A critical reappraisal of dietary practices in methylmalonic acidemia raises concerns about the safety of medical foods. Part 2: Cobalamin C deficiency. *Genetics in Medicine* 18(4):396–404.

Ney, D. M., S. G. Murali, B. M. Stroup, M. Nair, E. A. Sawin, F. Rohr, and H. L. Levy. 2017. Metabolomic changes demonstrate reduced bioavailability of tyrosine and altered metabolism of tryptophan via the kynurenine pathway with ingestion of medical foods in phenylketonuria. *Molecular Genetics and Metabolism* 121(2):96–103.

Parikh, S., A. Goldstein, M. K. Koenig, F. Scaglia, G. M. Enns, R. Saneto, I. Anselm, B. H. Cohen, M. J. Falk, C. Greene, A. L. Gropman, R. Haas, M. Hirano, P. Morgan, K. Sims, M. Tarnopolsky, J. L. Van Hove, L. Wolfe, and S. DiMauro. 2015. Diagnosis and management of mitochondrial disease: A consensus statement from the Mitochondrial Medicine Society. *Genetics in Medicine* 17(9):689–701.

Pinto, A., M. F. Almeida, P. C. Ramos, S. Rocha, A. Guimas, R. Ribeiro, E. Martins, A. Bandeira, A. MacDonald, and J. C. Rocha. 2017. Nutritional status in patients with phenylketonuria using glycomacropeptide as their major protein source. *European Journal of Clinical Nutrition* 71(10):1230–1234.

Singh, R. H., A. C. Cunningham, S. Mofidi, T. D. Douglas, D. M. Frazier, D. G. Hook, L. Jeffers, H. McCune, K. D. Moseley, S. Ogata, S. Pendyal, J. Skrabal, P. L. Splett, A. Stembridge, A. Wessel, and F. Rohr. 2016. Updated, web-based nutrition management guideline for PKU: An evidence and consensus based approach. *Molecular Genetics and Metabolism* 118(2):72–83.

Stroup, B. M., E. A. Sawin, S. G. Murali, N. Binkley, K. E. Hansen, and D. M. Ney. 2017. Amino acid medical foods provide a high dietary acid load and increase urinary excretion of renal net acid, calcium, and magnesium compared with glycomacropeptide medical foods in phenylketonuria. *Journal of Nutrition and Metabolism* 2017:1909101. doi: 10.1155/2017/1909101.

3

Disease-Induced Loss of Function and Tissue Regeneration

Session 3 was moderated by Alex Kemper, Chief of the Division of Ambulatory Pediatrics at the Nationwide Children's Hospital, and a Planning Committee member. In the first presentation Christopher Duggan, Director of the Center for Nutrition at the Boston Children's Hospital, discussed examples of gastrointestinal (GI) dysfunction and nutrient malabsorption in intestinal failure. The next speaker, Sarah Jane Schwarzenberg, Chief of Pediatric Gastroenterology, Hepatology, and Nutrition at the University of Minnesota Masonic Children's Hospital, also provided an overview of GI dysfunction and nutrient malabsorption, focusing on cystic fibrosis (CF). The third speaker was Dale Lee, Assistant Professor of Pediatrics at the Seattle Children's Hospital. He presented an overview of nutritional requirements for inflammatory bowel disease (IBD). In the following presentation, Martha Field, Assistant Professor in the Division of Nutritional Sciences at Cornell University, discussed blood–brain barrier dysfunction and resulting brain nutrient deficiencies. The final presentation, which covered macronutrient and micronutrient homeostasis in the setting of chronic kidney disease (CKD), was provided by Alp Ikizler, Professor of Medicine at the Vanderbilt University School of Medicine. A moderated panel discussion and question and answer session concluded the session.

EXAMPLES OF GASTROINTESTINAL DYSFUNCTION AND MALABSORPTION OF NUTRIENTS: INTESTINAL FAILURE[1]

Intestinal failure is characterized by a reduction of functional intestinal mass necessary for adequate digestion and absorption to meet nutrient, fluid, and growth requirements. By definition, Duggan explained, the condition requires specialized nutritional support through either the enteral or parenteral route. Intestinal failure has three physiological classifications: short bowel syndrome, GI motility disorders, and intestinal epithelial defects. Duggan stated that his presentation would focus mainly on surgical short bowel syndrome, a condition resulting from massive resection of portions of the GI tract.

Duggan noted that short bowel syndrome has been defined as intestinal loss due to acquired or congenital disease leading to dependence on parenteral nutrition for more than 90 days. He noted that this 90-day cutoff is admittedly arbitrary but seems to correlate with the occurrence of a number of side effects of long-term parenteral nutrition so is considered to be clinically reasonable. Some papers have used shorter cut-off times (e.g., 60 days) or anatomical definitions.

Duggan explained that until relatively recently, more than one-half of pediatric patients with short bowel syndrome either died or underwent multivisceral transplantation, which involves transplantation of three or more abdominal organs (Squires et al., 2012). As care of patients with intestinal failure has improved, the survival rate has continued to increase, to the point that some centers are publishing 90 percent or near 100 percent survival rates, even among those with chronic, refractory disease (Duggan and Jaksic, 2017).

Patients with intestinal failure have massive bowel loss or intestinal dysfunction which, depending on extent and location of resection, leads to malabsorption of all three classes of macronutrients and many micronutrients. Therefore, the mainstay of intestinal failure treatment, Duggan explained, is early and aggressive parenteral nutrition, with gradually increasing amounts of enteral nutrition as the bowel adapts after massive resection. Micronutrient supplementation is an important therapy as well. A number of medical and surgical therapies for underlying complications from intestinal failure are being developed, including new hormone analogs for glucagon-like peptide-2, surgical therapies that taper and lengthen the bowel, and multivisceral transplantation. The underlying and perhaps most effective therapy, however, remains supporting the body's natural process of intestinal adaptation (i.e., the process wherein residual bowel becomes more efficient at absorbing nutrients).

---

[1] This section summarizes information presented by Christopher Duggan.

In addition to the malabsorption of nutrients, complications of intestinal failure include liver disease and fat malabsorption due to pancreatic insufficiency. Duggan argued that intestinal failure-associated liver disease seems to be related largely to toxicity of additives in long-term parenteral nutrition, as opposed to nutrient deficiencies. These findings, he said, raise the issue of whether the route of administration of nutrients needs to be considered when determining nutrient requirements and toxicities.

Nutritional requirements in patients with intestinal failure are different from those of a healthy population. "Total" parenteral nutrition, however, is a misnomer, in that it does not meet all nutrient requirements. In addition, Duggan said, nutritional therapy for intestinal failure is a supportive, not curative, therapy per se (unless a patient has severe acute malnutrition or important micronutrient deficiencies). A retrospective review of children with intestinal failure at Boston Children's Hospital showed a high prevalence of various micronutrient deficiencies, even while the patient was receiving parenteral nutrition at least several days per week at a center that takes special care to maintain children on micronutrient supplementations as they are weaning from parenteral nutrition (Yang et al., 2011; see Figure 3-1).

Duggan went on to say that recommendations for pediatric parenteral nutrition intakes from groups such as the American Society for Parenteral and Enteral Nutrition have shifted over time depending on the nutrient under study, that these recommendations have often been based on expert opinion, and that they are often derived from clinical observations of nutrient deficiency states, and/or by extrapolation from adult or animal data.

Supporting data for different nutritional requirements for patients who are dependent on intravenous nutrition or transitioning from parenteral to enteral nutrition are limited and often derived from empiric observations, such as lack of weight gain or lack of height gain in children and infants, and laboratory data in others. Requirements for many nutrients have been demonstrated when the omission of important vital nutrients resulted in clinically apparent deficiencies. Data for conditionally essential nutrients in the context of intestinal malabsorption or dependence on parenteral nutrition are also weak. Glutamine supplementation offers a perfect example of these issues, Duggan explained. In this case, animal and other data on the requirement for glutamine in the study of GI diseases are quite voluminous, but when the nutrient was examined carefully in large randomized trials, no positive effect was seen from parenteral glutamine supplementation among premature infants.

Duggan concluded his presentation by noting that although patients with intestinal failure have taught the nutrition community a substantial

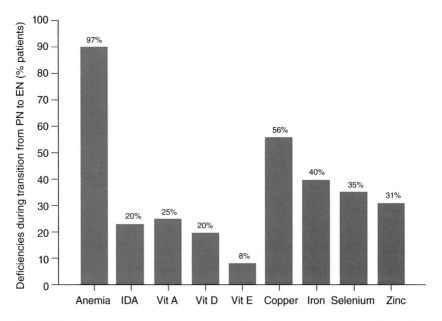

FIGURE 3-1 Prevalence of micronutrient deficiencies during parenteral nutrition weaning.
NOTE: EN = enteral nutrition; IDA = iron deficiency anemia; PN = parenteral nutrition.
SOURCES: As presented by Christopher Duggan, April 2, 2018; Yang et al., 2011. Reprinted from *Journal of Pediatrics*, volume 159, issue 1, Yang, C. F., D. Duro, D. Zurakowski, M. Lee, T. Jaksic, and C. Duggan, High prevalence of multiple micronutrient deficiencies in children with intestinal failure: A longitudinal study, pages 39–44, Copyright 2011, with permission from Elsevier. https://www.sciencedirect.com/journal/the-journal-of-pediatrics (accessed June 6, 2018).

amount about nutrient needs in health and disease, it is difficult to study nutrient needs in this condition because of the

- rarity of the condition;
- small size of infants and concomitant limited availability of blood and other biologic specimen volumes;
- lack of valid biomarkers for nutritional status;
- heterogeneity of intestinal absorptive capacity among subjects; and
- limited ability to perform cross-over studies because the majority of patients are growing children and are difficult to consider in steady state.

EXAMPLES OF GASTROINTESTINAL DYSFUNCTION AND MALABSORPTION OF NUTRIENTS: CYSTIC FIBROSIS[2]

CF occurs in about 1 in 3,500 individuals in the United States and Europe, and is one of the more common genetic diseases. It is caused by loss-of-function mutations in the cystic fibrosis transmembrane conductance regulator (CFTR) gene. Approximately 1,000 genetic mutations have been demonstrated in the CFTR gene. Many of them lead to clinical disease with variable consequences.

The CFTR protein mediates the secretion of chloride and bicarbonate as well as water across the epithelial layer. Loss of this function results in progressive obstructive lung disease that generally leads to death in the fourth decade. Management of CF generally involves maintaining pulmonary function and controlling infections.

In the United States, care for about 85 percent of CF patients is provided through Cystic Fibrosis Foundation care centers, which also includes a patient registry with data on infections, nutrition, liver disease, pulmonary function, and other information. These data allow care centers to compare survival, body mass index (BMI), 1-second forced expiratory volume, and many other aspects of CF.

Nutrition-Related Features of Cystic Fibrosis

Schwarzenberg explained that although CF is predominantly a lung disease, the disease also has the following significant impact on nutrition:

- People with CF require more calories than average because of increased pulmonary effort and chronic and recurrent inflammation. At the same time, they often have poor appetite and intake.
- People with CF often have abnormalities of motility, diminished sense of smell, abdominal pain and depression, malabsorption related to pancreatic insufficiency, and small bowel overgrowth. They also have a unique form of diabetes and a unique form of liver disease, each of which affects nutrition. CF-related diabetes affects about 50 percent of people with CF over the lifespan, mainly as the result of the loss of islet function in the pancreas.
- Most individuals with CF are pancreatic insufficient at birth, and 85 percent will be pancreatic insufficient by age 1. Clinicians try to offset this through pancreatic enzyme replacement therapy, but even at its most successful, this therapy allows patients to digest about 95 percent of the fat ingested.

---

[2] This section summarizes information presented by Sarah Jane Schwarzenberg.

- Chronic intestinal inflammation, a less well recognized problem than pancreatic insufficiency, often occurs. This leads to thick and dehydrated intestinal mucus and to bacterial growth against the intestinal lining. The resulting dysbiosis is exacerbated by the repeated antibiotic use, ending in intestinal lesions with symptoms such as diarrhea, bloating, nausea, abdominal pain, and distention.
- Intestinal bicarbonate in enterocytes and pancreas is decreased. This is important for absorption of fat (absorption of fat requires the production of mixed micelles with bile acids, and bile acids do not remain in solution at low pH) and for the activity of the enteric-coated pancreatic enzymes used today (they will not dissolve in acidic pHs).
- Patients with CF can develop a unique form of liver disease. This focal biliary fibrosis and multilobular cirrhosis, which can occur with or without portal hypertension, is the third leading cause of death in CF. The main issue for people with CF and nutrition is the reduction in the production of bile salts associated with liver disease.
- Dysbiosis results in intestinal dysmotility and gastroparesis. Gastroparesis affects about one-third of individuals with CF, resulting in nausea, early satiety, persistent dyspepsia, and abdominal pain.
- Sinus disease is also common in CF and manifests through nasal polyps that impair the sense of smell, contributing to the lack of appetite and thick retropharyngeal mucus.

Evidence since the 1980s has indicated that maintenance of weight greater than the 50th percentile for age and sex is associated with longer survival. Good nutritional management may result in an additional decade of life, which is quite significant in CF. For example, a prospective observational study using data from the Cystic Fibrosis Foundation registry (see Figure 3-2) showed that pulmonary function was much lower in CF patients with a weight-for-age percentile less than 10 percent at age 4. This outcome tracked through 18 years of life. The main takeaway, noted Schwarzenberg, is that clinicians should try to keep patients on the same weight-for-age percentile throughout life. Many healthy children grow on the 10th percentile, but CF patients must be at the 50th percentile or greater in order to achieve the longest life possible.

Cystic Fibrosis Nutrition Interventions

CF-specific nutritional interventions are driven by quality improvement projects and guidelines developed by the Cystic Fibrosis Foundation. It is well established that children who obtain newborn screening

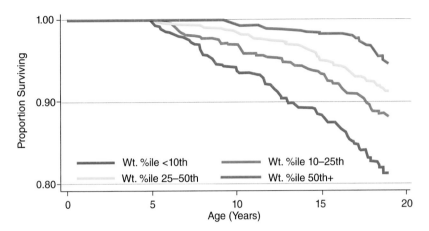

FIGURE 3-2 Survival in children with cystic fibrosis at various weight-for-age percentiles.
NOTE: Survival was highest in patients with better weight-for-age percentiles at 4 years of age.
SOURCES: As presented by Sarah Jane Schwarzenberg, April 2, 2018; Yen et al., 2013. Reprinted from *Journal of Pediatrics*, volume 162/issue 3, Yen, E. H., H. Quinton, and D. Borowitz, Better nutritional status in early childhood is associated with improved clinical outcomes and survival in patients with cystic fibrosis, pages 530–535, Copyright 2013, with permission from Elsevier. https://www.sciencedirect.com/journal/the-journal-of-pediatrics (accessed June 6, 2018).

and who are introduced to good nutrition before the age of 2 or 3 months have better health outcomes than children whose diagnosis is made even a short time later. Children are asked to eat a high-fat diet to increase calories, and to eat three meals and three snacks every day. Schwarzenberg noted that this is very hard for many patients. Patients are given water-miscible fat-soluble vitamin supplementation because they generally cannot adequately absorb ordinary vitamin supplements.

Schwarzenberg then briefly mentioned some interventions that improve the function of some gene mutations in CF. One in particular is ivacaftor, which makes gating mutations less injurious. These mutations occur in about 4 to 6 percent of people with CF, but people on ivacaftor experience improved lung function and reduced sweat chloride and they gain weight, perhaps due to the release of bicarbonate into the GI tract.

Research Gaps

Schwarzenberg admitted that the research gaps in CF and nutrition are numerous, but she noted that the following questions highlight key gaps:

- What is the cause of dysbiosis and dysmotility in CF, and how is it best managed?
- What is the appropriate fat type for people with CF to ensure adequate essential fatty acids without increasing inflammatory products?
- How should nutrition be addressed as patients age and new complications occur?
- What effect will new modulators of CFTR have on nutrition?

Schwarzenberg concluded her presentation by summarizing that in CF, better early childhood nutrition is associated with better height growth, better lung function, and improved survival into adulthood. However, optimal nutrition in CF is not a simple matter of increased calories. Clinicians must pay attention to a complex disordered matrix of digestion, absorption, and intestinal function, and that is really the challenge in this disease.

NUTRITIONAL REQUIREMENTS FOR INFLAMMATORY BOWEL DISEASE[3]

IBD is a chronic inflammatory condition with symptoms including abdominal pain, diarrhea, and blood in the stool, and systemic manifestations such as fever, body rashes, linear growth delay, and poor weight gain. IBD has two types. Crohn's disease involves any portion of the GI tract, from mouth to anus, and ulcerative colitis is confined to the colon. IBD arises in the setting of a genetic predisposition, but numerous environmental insults can occur to trigger a perpetuating cycle of inflammation. At least 200 known genes are associated with IBD risk, explained Lee. The known environmental risk factors include antibiotic exposures, certain dietary exposures, and infections. When these environmental exposures occur in the setting of a genetic risk, a breach of the epithelial barrier of the GI tract can occur. Translocation of microbial products may occur, which stimulates the immune system to react and develop an inflammatory reaction. The chronic inflammation in IBD can lead to complications, including scarring and infections in the GI tract and increased risk of intestinal cancers.

Lee stated that epidemiological studies have shown that diet and nutrients are important for IBD. Immigration studies also have implicated the role of environment and diet. In addition, it is known that exclusion diets can be effective in treating IBD. Although several risk factors (e.g., total saturated fat, total polyunsaturated fatty acids, omega-6 poly-

---

[3] This section summarizes information presented by Dale Lee.

unsaturated fatty acid, and meats) and protective dietary factors (e.g., fiber, fruits, vegetables, and omega-3 polyunsaturated fatty acids) have been identified, it is unclear whether these are actually risk and protective factors, or whether individuals at risk of developing IBD merely have different nutrient requirements.

Nutrient Deficiencies Associated with Inflammatory Bowel Disease

It is known that individuals with systemic inflammation and IBD have anorexia, so they have decreased global intake of macro- and micro-nutrients. Individuals with IBD also often have malabsorption and resultant diarrhea and deficiency of fat-soluble vitamins and zinc. Intestinal blood loss with IBD can lead to iron deficiency. The chronic systemic inflammation that occurs in IBD can lead to anemia and activated 1,25 hydroxy vitamin D deficiency. With Crohn's disease in particular, the most common area of IBD inflammation is the ileum, or the distal small bowel, and as a result, patients can develop vitamin B12 deficiencies.

Role of Nutrient Supplementation

In general, the current approach to treating IBD is to focus on controlling the active inflammation, which can help improve nutrient status. As an adjunct, supplementation with specific nutrients, such as vitamin D, iron, vitamin B12 injections, zinc, and a variety of other B vitamins, may be recommended.

Lee elaborated by discussing vitamin D and the risk of developing IBD, using the Harvard Nurses' Health Study to illustrate. Among study participants, the risk of developing Crohn's disease in the highest quartile of serum vitamin D appeared to be lower than for the lowest quartile. When a similar study was done analyzing for ulcerative colitis, investigators did not find significant associations, suggesting that Crohn's and ulcerative colitis, though both IBDs, have a different pathogenesis. Some trials that have explored the role of vitamin D supplementation in IBD have suggested that increased vitamin D is associated with a decreased risk of disease relapse, and in children, that markers of inflammation are reduced. In terms of iron deficiency, production of hepcidin, a protein produced by the liver that causes decreased uptake of iron from the GI tract and decreased mobilization of iron from the liver and spleen, can be induced in IBD.

Treatment

Switching gears, Lee described the strategies for treating IBD. The mainstream treatment is the use of immunosuppressive medications, such as corticosteroids, immunomodulators, and biological medications. In terms of nutritional therapy, exclusive enteral nutrition (EEN) therapy is a formula-based approach. A number of specific exclusion diets used for IBD have stimulated provocative, relatively large-scale studies.

Lee explained that EEN therapy for IBD involves consumption of a defined formula (by mouth, delivered by nasogastric tube, or delivered by a gastrostomy tube) that accounts for the patient's entire nutritional needs. Studies have demonstrated that the type of formula is not important, in that it can have intact protein or protein hydrolysate with different carbohydrate and fat content. The formula supplements calories and controls the inflammation in Crohn's disease. Studies in children with Crohn's have demonstrated that EEN is associated with about 80 percent induction of clinical remission. In one Italian study, comparing a group using EEN and controls, both groups achieved fairly good clinical remission rates (greater than 60 percent), but the EEN group had greater than 70 percent mucosal healing, whereas the corticosteroid group had only 30 percent mucosal healing (Borrelli et al., 2006). These results, noted Lee, suggest that the luminal delivery of nutrition was superior to broad immunosuppression of the corticosteroids.

Lee also described a second study, the PLEASE study, in which children with active Crohn's disease were divided into three groups—partial enteral nutrition, EEN, and a biological medication (Lee et al., 2015). The outcomes examined were clinical disease activity and fecal calprotectin, a surrogate marker of intestinal inflammation that can be measured in the stool. Results showed outcomes for the EEN group were clearly superior to the partial enteral nutrition group for both outcomes.

Elaborating on the point that appropriate delivery of nutrition is important, Lee noted that studies have looked at allowing nothing by mouth and delivering nutrition solely through the intravenous route. Results showed that for individuals with IBD, this approach would greatly benefit overall nutritional status but would not affect the eventual need for surgery for these patients. Clearly, Lee noted, the contents in the lumen of the GI tract are important to intestinal health. It is known, for example, that fiber is fermented to short-chain fatty acids and short-chain fatty acids provide an energy source to intestinal epithelial cells, and they also have a role in promoting immune tolerance.

Knowing that a formula-based treatment approach works, the logical next question, noted Lee, is whether food-based dietary therapy for IBD also works. A few food-based dietary approaches have been gaining in traction, including a specific carbohydrate diet, the Crohn's diseases exclusion diet, semi-vegetarian diets, and a variety of different anti-inflammatory diets. Each of these diets involves the restriction of certain food groups. The most commonly avoided food groups are bread and gluten and also "processed foods," a broad, poorly defined category. On the other hand, restricted diets are of some concern because they eliminate entire food groups from the diet, which can be problematic for nutritional adequacy and emotional well-being of individuals.

The specific carbohydrate diet, which was initially proposed as a dietary therapy for celiac disease, has an extremely broad following for a variety of different GI illnesses. However, rigorous studies need to be conducted to determine their usefulness in this context. Some studies, mostly case series, conducted on the effect of the specific carbohydrate diet on clinical disease activity indices as well as laboratory parameters suggest that patients experienced some improvement. To help answer some questions regarding the carbohydrate diets, the results of two ongoing large, multi-center trials will be helpful. An N-of-1 study with children is exploring the specific carbohydrate diet. (For more information on N-of-1 studies, see Nicholas Schork's presentation in Chapter 5.) In the adult arena, the University of Pennsylvania has designed a multi-center study looking at the specific carbohydrate diet versus the Mediterranean diet. This study will look at objective markers of inflammation, clinical disease activity, and the microbiome.

Complexities of Inflammatory Bowel Disease and Nutrients

Lee then summarized the following complexities with IBD and nutrients:

- Nutritional therapy is used differently for Crohn's and ulcerative colitis and the formula-based approach (i.e., EEN) is effective only for Crohn's disease.
- Genetic polymorphisms are known to be associated with the efficacy of the formula-based approach. The NOD2 gene is involved with bacterial product recognition. Polymorphisms of this gene have been associated with efficacy of EEN therapy.
- In active inflammation versus quiescent disease, vitamin D and iron may be processed differently. For vitamin D, individuals with active inflammation have a decreased parathyroid hormone activity and decreased 1-alpha-hydroxylation of 25-hydroxy vitamin D at the renal level.

Gaps in Knowledge

Finally, Lee noted the following gaps in current understanding about IBD and nutrition:

- The role of specific dietary components on IBD pathogenesis needs to be better elucidated. These components go beyond macro- and micronutrients to include food additives and products generated during cooking.
- Better methodologies, specifically biomarkers, are needed to assess dietary exposures.
- A better understanding of the interplay among diet, the intestinal microbiome, and the metabolome is needed, as these data will help inform individual-focused interventions.

BLOOD–BRAIN BARRIER DYSFUNCTION AND RESULTING BRAIN NUTRIENT DEFICIENCIES[4]

Field began her remarks by showing a figure that illustrates the relationships between disease etiology, physiological impact on nutrients and function, and impact on human nutrition and on biomarkers (see Figure 3-3).

Field noted that the framework shown in the figure provides the context to examine how several disease-related factors, including inflammation, genetic predisposition, autoimmunity, and mitochondrial dysfunction, specifically affect the blood–brain barrier (BBB) and then influence cerebral folate deficiency (CFD).

Cerebrospinal fluid (CSF) serves as a nourishing fluid for the brain and a way to remove waste products. The epithelial and endothelial barriers, which are components of the BBB, are critical for maintaining brain nutritional status as they serve to concentrate nutrients through a variety of mechanisms (e.g., vitamin C and folate are concentrated fourfold in the CSF relative to the serum; many B vitamins are concentrated, some as much as 50-fold). BBB function, however, declines as a result of disease (e.g., Alzheimer's disease, multiple sclerosis, human immunodeficiency virus infection), inflammation, or aging. This dysfunction can occur due to a loss of transport protein expression or erosion of the tight junctions in the BBB that prevent nutrients or other molecules from leaking out of the brain.

CFD, which can result from BBB dysfunction, affects the metabolic functions of folate within the brain. Folates carry and chemically activate one-carbon units for biosynthetic reactions. More specifically, folate is needed to synthesize purines and thymidylate and for the remethylation of homocysteine to methionine. Methionine is a precursor of S-adenosylmethionine, which is required for methylation of deoxyribonucleic acid (DNA), and histones, and in synthesis of neural transmitters. Folate is transported across the BBB

---

[4] This section summarizes information presented by Martha Field.

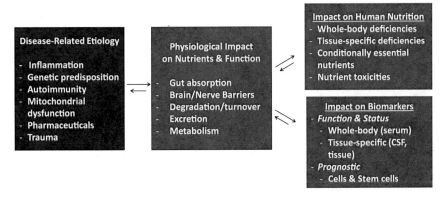

FIGURE 3-3 Influence of disease on whole-body nutrient status and tissue-specific nutrient status.
NOTE: CSF = cerebrospinal fluid.
SOURCE: As presented by Martha Field, April 2, 2018.

to the CSF at the choroid plexus by receptor-mediated endocytosis, and this process is mediated by folate receptor alpha in an adenosine triphosphate (ATP)-dependent manner. Because of the difference in folate concentration in the CSF relative to the blood, CSF folate levels indicate brain folate status independent of indicators of whole-body folate status.

Inborn Errors of Metabolism and Cerebral Folate Deficiency

Field noted that a number of studies demonstrate that individuals with inborn errors of metabolism in the folate receptor or with genetic disorders that cause mitochondrial DNA dysfunction—in other words, either a mutation in the receptor or a loss of ability to generate ATP—develop CFD and exhibit CSF folate levels much lower than normal (around 100 nanomolar). Successful intervention for CFD requires high-dose folinic acid, a reduced form of folate. Folic acid, a synthetic form of folate, is highly bioavailable and chemically stable but not as effective as folinic acid or methyl folate (a B vitamin form in fruits and vegetables) at improving CSF folate levels, possibly due to the ability of folic acid to bind tightly to the receptor, impairing transport of methyl folate across the BBB. In fact, at the very high folic acid doses that are shown to be effective in addressing CFD, folic acid can be associated with some toxicity.

Field noted that the relationship between impairments in whole body folate status and brain disease or, more specifically, depression, have been recognized by authoritative bodies, including the American Psychiatric Association, the Institute of Medicine, and the World Health Organization

(APA, 2010; de Benoist, 2008; IOM, 1998). She then went on to explain how this association between whole body folate status and depression parallels with inborn errors of metabolism and a tissue-specific nutrient deficiency. A genetic component to the link between CFD or between low folate status and depression exists. One common genetic variant, a single nucleotide change in the *MTHFR* gene (*MTHFR* C677T), affects the functioning of folate-mediated one-carbon metabolism and folate status. Neural tube defect risk is doubled for carriers of the TT genotype, which is also associated with increased risk of miscarriage. Interestingly, in folate-sufficient adults, the TT genotype is protective against colon cancer.

Because of its effect on lowering folate status, the *MTHFR* T allele has been associated with increased risk of developing both depression and schizophrenia, and up to 70 percent of patients with either depression or schizophrenia have some form of the polymorphism (i.e., one or two T alleles). On the other hand, major depressive disorder, projected to be the second leading global disease burden by 2020, is responsive to standard medication in less than one-half of all patients. The etiology of major depressive disorder is poorly understood but is likely to involve a complex interplay of sensitivities to stressors and alterations in metabolic pathways. Some evidence suggests that BBB integrity is compromised in depressed patients. Several informative clinical trials to examine folate-related treatments for depression suggest that both the form of folate and the dose influence the efficacy for folate in improving depression-related outcomes (Alpert et al., 2002; Papakostas et al., 2012, 2014). When describing results from the trials, Field emphasized that the doses used are very different than requirements in healthy individuals, by more than an order of magnitude. She also noted that although the origins of CFD are very different than those caused by inborn errors of metabolism, the treatments that result in clinical improvement are essentially the same.

Field then provided the following summary of her presentation:

- Brain-specific folate deficiency can occur in the absence of whole body deficiency in inborn errors of metabolism and in adult disease, although whole body deficiency could exacerbate the condition.
- BBB folate transport defects can be overcome with high levels of folate. Folate form or composition matters for efficacy. Reduced folates are efficacious; folic acid is not.
- This evidence clearly indicates a different nutritional requirement in these conditions than for healthy population.
- The disease states are responsive to intervention, but some individuals are responders and others are not. There does seem to be evidence of dose response.

- Understanding these relationships requires an understanding of biomarkers and rigorous, well-designed controlled trials.

Field concluded her presentation by reiterating that several nutrients, not only folate, are concentrated within the brain, and that little is currently known about how these nutrients are affected by disruptions in BBB activity. It is also not well understood whether repairing the barrier can reverse the nutritional deficiency and/or whether restoring brain nutrient levels can augment BBB repair.

MACRO- AND MICRONUTRIENT HOMEOSTASIS IN THE SETTING OF CHRONIC KIDNEY DISEASE[5]

In contrast to most of the conditions discussed in previous presentations, Ikizler stated that kidney disease is very common. About 20 million individuals in the United States have CKD. The mortality rate in the setting of end-stage renal disease is about 20 percent per year. Ikizler also noted that, as with any other chronic disease state, nutrition is one of the most important, if not the most important, predictors of outcomes.

Turning his attention to the nutrition aspects of chronic kidney disease, Ikizler noted that protein energy wasting (PEW) is highly prevalent in this patient population (about 12 to 18 percent of all patients with CKD not yet on maintenance dialysis and 30 to 50 percent for patients on dialysis). Kidney disease leads to PEW for multiple reasons. Ikizler observed that in developed countries, PEW, sarcopenia, wasting syndrome, and malnutrition predispose patients to significant complications that are associated with PEW, such as infection, cardiovascular disease, and frailty, that in aggregate or individually put CKD patients at increased mortality risk.

Evidence of Unique Nutritional Requirements in Chronic Kidney Disease

A number of studies have established the need for more or less of the nutrients that are usually given to healthy individuals[6] in various disease states, including CKD (see Table 3-1).

In describing this table, Ikizler noted that protein requirements are significantly altered at different stages of kidney disease and different from the needs of the general population. Dietary requirements (e.g., sup-

---

[5] This section summarizes information presented by Alp Ikizler.
[6] For Dietary Reference Intake (DRI) values, see http://nationalacademies.org/HMD/Activities/Nutrition/SummaryDRIs/DRI-Tables.aspx (accessed June 6, 2018).

TABLE 3-1 Summary of Nutrient Requirements in Chronic Kidney Disease

	Non-Dialysis CKD	Hemodialysis	Peritoneal Dialysis
Energy	30–35 kcal/kg/day	35 kcal/kg/day	35 kcal/kg/day including kcal from dialysate
Protein	0.6–0.8 g/kg/day Illness 1.0 g/kg	>1.2 g/kg/day	>1.2 g/kg/day Peritonitis >1.5 g/kg
Sodium	80–100 mmol/day	80–100 mmol/day	80–100 mmol/day
Potassium	<1 mmol/kg if elevated	<1 mmol/kg if elevated	Not usually an issue
Phosphorus	800–1,000 mg and binders if elevated	800–1,000 mg and binders if elevated	800–1,000 mg and binders if elevated

NOTE: CKD = chronic kidney disease.
SOURCES: As presented by Alp Ikizler, April 2, 2018; Cano et al., 2006; Fouque et al., 2007; NKF/KDOQI, 2000, 2002.

plementation, limitations, or restrictions) must be determined based on each patient's background and level of kidney function. Studies suggest that higher protein intakes, greater than 1.0 or 1.2 grams per kilogram per day, could be associated with progression of kidney disease. In contrast, patients with end-stage renal disease experience the syndrome of protein wasting and they have substantial need for additional protein intake. Other evidence suggests that patients with obesity who have end-stage renal disease do better than patients with normal weight. In the setting of CKD, however, patients with obesity actually experience much faster progression of their kidney disease than patients with normal weight.

Nutrition Issues in Chronic Kidney Disease

Ikizler continued by explaining that CKD has three nutrition issues of relevance: changes in requirements for protein intake, hemodialysis-associated catabolism, and the effect of inflammation and how it influences the metabolic profile of people with kidney disease.

He reminded workshop participants that the hallmark of uremia (or uremic syndrome, that is, urea in the blood due to an excess of amino acid and protein metabolism into end-products in the blood that would be normally excreted in the urine) is anorexia. The initiation of dialysis in CKD patients with uremia occurs when they became anorexic and cannot eat adequately. This decrease in nutrient intake, especially protein, progresses as the glomerular filtration rate (GFR) goes down from greater than 60 to 30 or less. The initiation of dialysis reverses this problem to some extent, but dialysis in itself is inadequate to replace original kidney function, and the initial improvement subsides over the course of 3 to 4 years. Restricting protein in earlier stages of kidney disease limits the amount of protein being metabolized and the uremic toxins that are produced through this process are decreased, which results in less nausea and other uremic symptoms.

Another problem with maintenance dialysis is that in addition to filtering out undesirable molecules, it also eliminates other small molecules, such as essential amino acids. The resulting diminished amino acid pool leads to increased catabolism and decreased protein synthesis, which results in robust net catabolism. Results from a study that examined protein turnover using stable isotopes show a significant drop in the protein synthesis and a significant increase in protein breakdown, resulting in an almost doubling of the net catabolic process (Ikizler et al., 2002).

Dialysis itself causes a loss of protein and the catabolic process continues after dialysis is completed, probably because the complement system and subsequently the inflammatory pathway (interleukin [IL]-6 and other inflammatory cytokines) become activated. In kidney disease, the average C-reactive protein or IL-6 concentrations are threefold or higher than for healthy individuals, leading to poor outcomes.

Responsiveness of Chronic Kidney Disease to Nutritional Intervention

CKD responds to specific nutritional interventions, Ikizler explained, but like many other aspects of this disease, it is complex. Limiting protein intake to less than 0.6 g/kg/day is desirable in CKD for the following reasons:

- It delays the initiation of uremic syndrome.
- It preserves kidney function by decreasing the load on remaining nephrons.
- It improves proteinuria/albuminuria.
- It improves metabolic profiles (i.e., decreased inflammation and oxidative stress, and increased insulin sensitivity) of CKD patients.

In fact, protein restriction may delay GFR decline by an average of 0.5 mL/min/year. However, Ikizler stated, the opposite is true for dialysis patients. That is, providing additional protein to individuals during dialysis at the setting with catabolic effect can completely reverse the process and initiate a robust anabolic response (Deger et al., 2017). A number of randomized controlled trials (RCTs) suggest that benefits to the intermediate surrogate outcomes of nutritional state, such as serum albumin, pre-albumin, body weight, lean body mass, bone density, and physical function, occur with protein supplementation. A recently completed study examined the effects of nutritional supplementation using a dual glucose-amino acid clamp procedure on changes in muscle protein signaling (Gamboa et al., 2016). In contrast to healthy controls, who showed an anabolic response, dialysis patients had no response. An examination under electron microscopy showed significant problems in the muscle tissue mitochondria that limits the full benefits of this nutritional supplementation in the setting of CKD. No information is available from RCTs on fat intake in the setting of CKD. Current recommendations follow those for the general population: low consumption of saturated fat and possible inclusion of omega-3 fatty acids. In terms of vitamins, the recommendation is that people with kidney disease should pay attention to intake of water-soluble vitamins because they are usually lost in dialysis, even though no evidence suggests that stores of these vitamins are extremely depleted. On the other hand, care must be taken with fat-soluble vitamins because they accumulate in the setting of kidney disease, especially vitamin A. Usually only vitamin D is supplemented. No information is available regarding trace elements in this context.

Gaps in Knowledge

Ikizler ended his presentation with a very brief roundup of current gaps in knowledge, including

- specific role of uremic toxins and the human microbiome;
- how to improve the dialysis process;
- optimal level of supplementation;
- the role of anabolic or anti-catabolic strategies; and
- obesity in CKD.

MODERATED PANEL DISCUSSION AND Q&A

Kemper initiated the discussion with a question to Duggan about whether it would ever be possible to have a scientific approach to determining what supplements an individual with intestinal failure needs. For example, would it be possible to take into account factors such as a patient's age, weight, how much residual bowel they have left, and comorbidities and determine a formula to figure out how much of these various nutrients they need? Duggan replied that that kind of prognostic equation would require much larger sample sizes and detailed intake data than are currently available but that it is a useful question to ponder.

On a question related to the response to nutrients in short bowel syndrome, when the metabolic homeostasis has been altered because of tissue loss, Duggan responded that a common etiology of gut resection in neonates is necrotizing enterocolitis, wherein resection preferentially occurs in the ileum and colon, which is exactly where intestinal L cells secrete glucagon peptide 2. An analog of this peptide has shown promise in adults but only limited data are available in children. Thinking more broadly, Duggan stated that the issue of whether the malabsorption of various nutrients can have a deleterious effect on intestinal adaptation is a little less clear. Although animal models have shown that vitamin A deficiency, for instance, reduces epithelial turnover, Duggan has not seen any data to suggest that high-dose vitamin A improves intestinal adaptation. Zinc is an important trace element as well for intestinal adaptation, but the animal model suggesting that profound zinc deficiency leads to decreased adaptation has not been well addressed in human trials, to his knowledge. Duggan also commented that some animal data suggest that bacterial overgrowth seems to relate to non-alcoholic fatty liver disease, acknowledging that valid methods to diagnose bacterial overgrowth in humans has been the main conundrum there.

Kemper noted a number of common elements, including the importance of determining not only the right nutrient or supplement to give but considering the right form and delivery system, and the important effect that inflammation seems to have on special nutritional requirements. Although levels of substances are generally measured in blood, plasma, or serum, levels in tissues are what is really desired. However, some tissues, such as brain, are difficult to sample. Field replied that the starting point with respect to tissues that are difficult to sample are mechanistic studies in animal models that provide a good understanding of the biology followed by studies of surrogate biomarkers.

Special Nutrient Requirements for
Metabolic Problems Not Directly Involving a Nutrient

An enquiry was raised on whether it is possible to have a special nutrient requirement in a metabolic problem that does not directly involve a nutrient. That is, can one just account for an absorption problem, or is there another way of thinking about the special nutrient requirement as it is affected by the metabolic state? Schwarzenberg replied that at least for CF the problem is more complex than just malabsorption. Although it is important management in CF to take into account the digestive and absorptive matrix abnormalities in the GI, nutrients are also being affected by the CFTR abnormality itself and by inflammation.

Ikizler addressed a related question regarding the role of inflammation in the diseases discussed during this session. From the kidney disease perspective, controversy exists over whether inflammation is the root cause of death in kidney disease patients. Although this can be determined only by examining the effect of anti-inflammatory interventions in the target outcome, he admitted that these studies are extremely complex because of the many outcomes involved that are interrelated and that might influence other outcomes or the disease process as a whole.

Evidence on Nutritional Factors That Trigger or Help the Disease Process

To a question related to whether any evidence exists that separates nutritional factors that trigger the disease versus those involved in treating or managing the disease, Lee responded that the evidence about risk and protective factors comes from large epidemiological studies that do not provide high-quality, detailed assessment of dietary data. The epidemiological studies cited in his presentation probably reflect both risk and protective factors and are probably pertinent for inception of disease and treatment. Lee added that when people think about nutrients, they generally think of the classically described macronutrients and micronutrients. However, food products consumed today include many other components that are not classified as nutrients and that need to be better understood.

The importance of studying not just single nutrients but patterns of dietary intake and how foods interact with each other was also raised. Schwarzenberg added that the dimension of time is also important to consider. An acute problem may be resolved, but the underlying pathologic process may continue for some time.

Conversion of Folate

A question was raised regarding the metabolic or environmental difficulties in the conversion of folate to folinic acid. Field replied that the fact that conversion of folic acid to the reduced form is saturable makes it very hard to get the high blood folate levels (above the Tolerable Upper Intake Level) needed to overcome the energetic barrier. These high levels cause GI toxicity and nephrotoxicity. However, Field continued, even at these high levels she would not consider folate to be a drug, because the nutrient requirement is a result of the disease itself (e.g., inflammation or Alzheimer's disease) and the breakdown of the BBB.

Effect of Nutritional Therapies on Cellular Composition of the Gut

The panel was asked whether any of the nutritional therapies for the conditions discussed during the session actually change the cellular composition of the intestine, for example goblet cell concentrations. According to Lee, studies have shown that changing the diet dramatically causes alterations in the microbiome as well as improvement in inflammation, although the exact causality is not easy to decipher. Ikizler noted that some ongoing research in CKD patients is also showing changes in the gut that may be due to inflammation or uremic toxins. The discussion continued with a question about whether it was possible to formulate a food matrix that contains specific functional proteins, pectins, or other components that interact with the microbiome to develop short-chain fatty acids for certain conditions. Lee responded that this is a critically important issue, and work is under way to better understand pathophysiology and how dietary changes affect the microbiome and how that microbiome interacts with the healthy host versus the inflamed diseased host.

Protein Dietary Reference Intakes and Chronic Kidney Disease

A comment was made on how potential increases in protein Dietary Reference Intakes might affect prevention of CKD in a population with a high prevalence of overweight or obesity.[7] This is an important dilemma, Ikizler replied, illustrating the balance between recommendations for the public when many people in that population have conditions, or risk factors for conditions, that would necessitate more tailored nutrition recommendations. Ikizler stated that in the era of precision medicine, individuals must be considered rather than just creating a generalized one-size-fits-all approach. There was general agreement among panel members that reducing calories overall and maintaining an appropriate distribution of macronutrients would be sufficient for individuals with obesity who might be at risk of diabetes or other chronic diseases.

Defining Malnutrition

The panel was asked to comment on how the lack of a definition of malnutrition hampers the ability to think about special nutrient requirements. Schwarzenberg responded that she was not certain that an overarching definition that would describe malnutrition in every chronic disease or every major disease is possible. Lee added that some very general

---

[7] For DRI values, see http://nationalacademies.org/HMD/Activities/Nutrition/Summary DRIs/DRI-Tables.aspx (accessed June 6, 2018).

criteria are available to diagnose malnutrition, such as weight for length Z scores, BMI Z scores, and weight loss over time. Astute clinicians and dieticians thinking about the appropriate trajectory for children will be needed in efforts to identify malnutrition and appropriate supplementation. Understanding the disease process is also critical.

REFERENCES

Alpert, J. E., D. Mischoulon, G. E. Rubenstein, K. Bottonari, A. A. Nierenbert, and M. Fava. 2002. Folinic acid (Leucovorin) as an adjunctive treatment for SSRI-refractory depression. *Annals of Clinical Psychiatry* 14(1):33–38.

APA (American Psychiatric Association). 2010. *Practice guideline for the treatment of patients with major depressive disorder.* Washington, DC: American Psychiatric Association.

Borrelli, O., L. Cordischi, M. Cirulli, M. Paganelli, V. Labalestra, S. Uccini, P. M. Russo, and S. Cucchiara. 2006. Polymeric diet alone versus corticosteroids in the treatment of active pediatric Crohn's disease: A randomized controlled open-label trial. *Clinical Gastroenterology amd Hepatology* 4(6):744–753.

Cano, N., E. Fiaccadori, P. Tesinsky, G. Toigo, W. Druml, DGEM (German Society for Nutritional Medicine), M. Kuhlmann, H. Mann, W. H. Horl, and ESPEN (European Society for Parenteral and Enteral Nutrition). 2006. ESPEN Guidelines on Enteral Nutrition: Adult renal failure. *Clinical Nutrition* 25(2):295–310.

de Benoist, B. 2008. Conclusions of a WHO technical consultation on folate and vitamin B12 deficiencies. *Food and Nutrition Bulletin* 29(2 Suppl.):S238–S244.

Deger, S. M., A. M. Hung, J. L. Gamboa, E. D. Siew, C. D. Ellis, C. Booker, F. Sha, H. Li, A. Bian, T. G. Stewart, R. Zent, W. E. Mitch, N. N. Abumrad, and T. A. Ikizler. 2017. Systemic inflammation is associated with exaggerated skeletal muscle protein catabolism in maintenance hemodialysis patients. *JCI Insight* 2(22):e95185.

Duggan, C. P., and T. Jaksic. 2017. Pediatric intestinal failure. *New England Journal of Medicine* 377(7):666–675.

Fouque, D., M. Vennegoor, P. Ter Wee, C. Wanner, A. Basci, B. Canaud, P. Haage, K. Konner, J. Kooman, A. Martin-Malo, L. Pedrini, F. Pizzarelli, J. Tattersall, J. Tordoir, and R. Vanholder. 2007. EBPG guideline on nutrition. *Nephrology Dialysis Transplantation* 22(Suppl. 2):ii45–ii87.

Gamboa, J. L., F. T. Billings, M. T. Bojanowski, L. A. Gilliam, C. Yu, B. Roshanravan, L. J. Roberts, J. Himmelfarb, T. A. Ikizler, and N. J. Brown. 2016. Mitochondrial dysfunction and oxidative stress in patients with chronic kidney disease. *Physiological Reports* 4(9):e12780.

Ikizler, T. A., L. B. Pupim, J. R. Brouillette, D. K. Levenhagen, K. Farmer, R. M. Hakim, and P. J. Flakoll. 2002. Hemodialysis stimulates muscle and whole body protein loss and alters substrate oxidation. *American Journal of Physiology-Endocrinology and Metabolism* 282(1):E107–E116.

IOM (Institute of Medicine). 1998. *Dietary Reference Intakes for thiamin, riboflavin, niacin, vitamin B6, folate, vitamin B12, pantothenic acid, biotin, and choline.* Washington, DC: National Academy Press.

Lee, D., R. N. Baldassano, A. R. Otley, L. Albenberg, A. M. Griffiths, C. Compher, E. Z. Chen, H. Li, E. Gilroy, L. Nessel, A. Grant, C. Chehoud, F. D. Bushman, G. D. Wu, and J. D. Lewis. 2015. Comparative effectiveness of nutritional and biological therapy in North American children with active Crohn's disease. *Inflammatory Bowel Diseases* 21(8):1786–1793.

NKF/KDOQI (National Kidney Foundation/Kidney Disease Outcomes Quality Initiative). 2000. *KDOQI Clinical Practice Guidelines for nutrition in chronic renal failure.* http://kidneyfoundation.cachefly.net/professionals/KDOQI/guidelines_nutrition/doqi_nut.html (accessed May 14, 2018).

NKF/KDOQI. 2002. *Clinical Practice Guidelines for chronic kidney disease: Evaluation, classification and stratification.* https://www.kidney.org/sites/default/files/docs/ckd_evaluation_classification_stratification.pdf (accessed May 11, 2018).

Papakostas, G. I., R. C. Shelton, J. M. Zajecka, B. Etemad, K. Rickels, A. Clain, L. Baer, E. D. Dalton, G. R. Sacco, D. Schoenfeld, M. Pencina, A. Meisner, T. Bottiglieri, E. Nelson, D. Mischoulon, J. E. Alpert, J. G. Barbee, S. Zisook, and M. Fava. 2012. L-methylfolate as adjunctive therapy for SSRI-resistant major depression: Results of two randomized, double-blind, parallel-sequential trials. *American Journal of Psychiatry* 169(12):1267–1274.

Papakostas, G. I., R. C. Shelton, J. M. Zajecka, T. Bottiglieri, J. Roffman, C. Cassiello, S. M. Stahl, and M. Fava. 2014. Effect of adjunctive L-methylfolate 15 mg among inadequate responders to SSRIs in depressed patients who were stratified by biomarker levels and genotype: Results from a randomized clinical trial. *Journal of Clinical Psychiatry* 75(8):855–863.

Squires, R. H., C. Duggan, D. H. Teitelbaum, P. W. Wales, J. Balint, R. Venick, S. Rhee, D. Sudan, D. Mercer, J. A. Martinez, B. A. Carter, J. Soden, S. Horslen, J. A. Rudolph, S. Kocoshis, R. Superina, S. Lawlor, T. Haller, M. Kurs-Lasky, S. H. Belle, and the Pediatric Intestinal Failure Consortium. 2012. Natural history of pediatric intestinal failure: Initial report from the Pediatric Intestinal Failure Consortium. *Journal of Pediatrics* 161(4):723–728.

Yang, C. F., D. Duro, D. Zurakowski, M. Lee, T. Jaksic, and C. Duggan. 2011. High prevalence of multiple micronutrient deficiencies in children with intestinal failure: A longitudinal study. *Journal of Pediatrics* 159(1):39–44.

Yen, E. H., H. Quinton, and D. Borowitz. 2013. Better nutritional status in early childhood is associated with improved clinical outcomes and survival in patients with cystic fibrosis. *Journal of Pediatrics* 162(3):530–535.

4

Disease-Induced Deficiency and Conditionally Essential Nutrients in Disease

S ession 4 was moderated by Bernadette Marriott, Professor in the Departments of Medicine and Psychiatry at the Medical University of South Carolina and a Planning Committee Member. In the first presentation, Claudia R. Morris, Associate Professor of Pediatrics and Emergency Medicine at the Emory University School of Medicine, discussed arginine as a conditionally essential nutrient, using sickle cell anemia and surgery as case examples. The second presenter was Angus Scrimgeour, a nutritional biochemist in the Military Nutrition Division at the U.S. Army Research Institute of Environmental Medicine. His presentation focused on pathophysiological mechanisms and potential nutrient needs in traumatic brain injury (TBI). In the third presentation, Jesse Gregory, Professor of Food Science and Human Nutrition at the University of Florida discussed the impact on nutrient requirements of metabolic turnover, inflammation, and redistribution. The session closed with a moderated panel discussion and question and answer session with workshop participants.

ARGININE AS AN EXAMPLE OF A CONDITIONALLY ESSENTIAL NUTRIENT: SICKLE CELL ANEMIA AND SURGERY[1]

Morris began her remarks by defining conditionally essential amino acids as amino acids that become indispensable under stress and critical illness when the capacity of endogenous synthesis is surpassed. Arginine

---

[1] This section summarizes information presented by Claudia Morris.

63

is one such amino acid, and Morris said that she would discuss sickle cell disease as an example of a condition that is associated with an acquired arginine deficiency.

What Is Arginine?

Morris explained that arginine is synthesized through the intestinal–renal axis and becomes essential under conditions of stress. It is found naturally in the diet; meat, dairy, seafood, nuts, and even watermelon are good sources. Arginine is a nutritional supplement with low toxicity and is the obligate substrate for nitric oxide production, a potent vasodilator that is important in regulating blood pressure. Arginine is converted to nitric oxide through the actions of enzymes, the nitric oxide synthases (NOSs). In addition to regulating vasodilatory tone, arginine also has an effect on platelet aggregation and in the immune response. It is a signaling molecule and can have some antioxidant effects. Arginine is also the substrate for arginase, an important enzyme in the urea cycle. This enzyme has two mammalian isoforms, arginase 1, which is cytosolic, and arginase 2, which is mitochondrial. Arginase is present in most cell types, including the red blood cell. Arginase is also upregulated in inflammation induced by cytokines, and ultimately competes with NOS for its common substrate of arginine. In the presence of arginase, arginine is converted to ornithine and urea. Ornithine and arginine use the same amino acid transporter, CAT-1 and CAT-2, so when ornithine levels rise, cellular uptake of arginine is inhibited, depending on how high the ornithine levels are. This could ultimately translate to decreased arginine and nitric oxide bioavailability. This means, said Morris, that arginine bioavailability cannot be derived by looking only at plasma arginine because other factors come into play, such as the presence of other amino acids that compete for intracellular transport.

Morris then showed a slide summarizing the arginine metabolome (see Figure 4-1). In many conditions of inflammation NOS is upregulated, yet paradoxically, nitric oxide production is decreased. It is known from the sickle cell mouse model that NOS, although it is upregulated, does not function properly and it can become uncoupled, where it produces superoxide in lieu of nitric oxide. This results in a dysfunctional arginine-to-nitric oxide pathway. This leads to substrate competition from arginase, which converts arginine to ornithine and pushes down the proliferative pathway to create prolines and polyamines. This is a pathway toward vascular smooth muscle proliferation, airway remodeling, and lung fibrosis. These structural changes are seen in the lungs of patients who develop pulmonary hypertension, a common comorbidity in sickle cell disease.

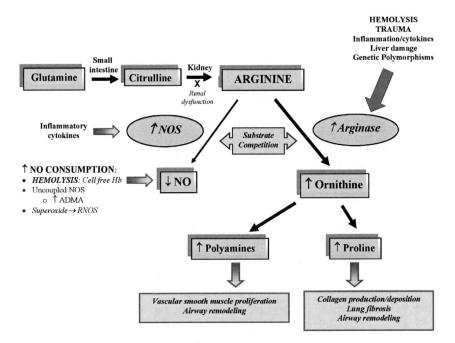

FIGURE 4-1 The arginine metabolome.

NOTES: Dietary glutamine serves as a precursor for the de novo production of arginine through the citrulline–arginine pathway. Arginine is synthesized endogenously from citrulline primarily via the intestinal–renal axis. Arginase and nitric oxide synthase (NOS) compete for arginine, their common substrate. In sickle cell disease and trauma, bioavailability of arginine and nitric oxide (NO) is decreased by several mechanisms linked to hemolysis, oxidative stress, and/or inflammation. Endothelial dysfunction resulting from NO depletion and increased levels of the downstream products of ornithine metabolism (poly-amines and proline) likely contribute to the pathogenesis of lung injury, fibrosis, and pulmonary hypertension commonly seen in sickle cell disease. This disease paradigm has implications for all hemolytic processes. Red arrows denote the influence of hemolysis and inflammation on the arginine–NO pathway and the downstream consequences in the lungs. ADMA = asymmetric dimethylarginine; Hb = hemoglobin; NO = nitric oxide; NOS = nitric oxide synthase; RNOS = reactive nitrogen oxide species.

SOURCES: As presented by Claudia Morris, April 2, 2018; Morris, 2008. Republished with permission of the American Society of Hematology. From Mechanisms of vasculopathy in sickle cell disease and thalassemia, Morris, C. R., 2008: 177–185. Permission conveyed through Copyright Clearance Center, Inc.

Morris noted that glutamine just received approval from the U.S. Food and Drug Administration (FDA) in the treatment of sickle cell disease due to its ability to decrease frequency of pain and acute chest syndrome. Thinking about arginine bioavailability, Morris noted that her group has coined the term "global arginine bioavailability ratio," a biomarker that correlates to important clinical outcomes and reflects arginine over the ratio of ornithine plus citrulline. This construct takes into account the impact of arginase, the impact on elevated ornithine levels and intracellular transport, and the effects of renal dysfunction as well as plasma arginine levels.

Sickle Cell Disease

Sickle cell disease is an autosomal recessive disease of the red blood cells that results in hemoglobin polymerization leading to a cascade of events that eventually cause decreased blood flow, tissue hypoxemia, and acute and chronic end organ damage in every organ system.

Eight percent of African Americans carry the sickle trait, explained Morris, and 1 out of 400 African Americans in the United States, or approximately 100,000 U.S. individuals, have sickle cell disease. Although it is considered an orphan disease in the United States because it affects fewer than 200,000 individuals, it affects millions of individuals worldwide.

Morris stated that a number of mechanisms of vasculopathy operate in sickle cell disease, with the depletion of nitric oxide taking center stage (see Figure 4-2).

Normally safely encapsulated within the red blood cell, the contents of the red blood cell break apart and are freed into circulation when hemolysis occurs (lactate dehydrogenase, found within the red blood cell freed into plasma during hemolysis, reflects the hemolytic rate and is a good biomarker of the hemolytic sub-phenotype of sickle cell disease). When the hemoglobin is freed into circulation, it rapidly consumes nitric oxide. The red cell also contains arginase, which when released during hemolysis rapidly consumes the obligate substrate for nitric oxide production. As the arginine level drops, the body reaches a threshold level below which NOS uncouples and produces superoxide in lieu of nitric oxide, further consuming nitric oxide and adding to the milieu of oxidative stress. Data from a large cohort of patients with sickle cell disease show the results from this cascade of events (Morris et al., 2005a). The clinical manifestations of hemolysis and decreased arginine-nitric oxide bioavailability include increased risk of stroke, renal insufficiency, priapism, leg ulcers, pulmonary hypertension, and possibly asthma.

Morris and her group investigated whether increasing arginase levels would ease the pulmonary hypertension. After 5 days of oral supple-

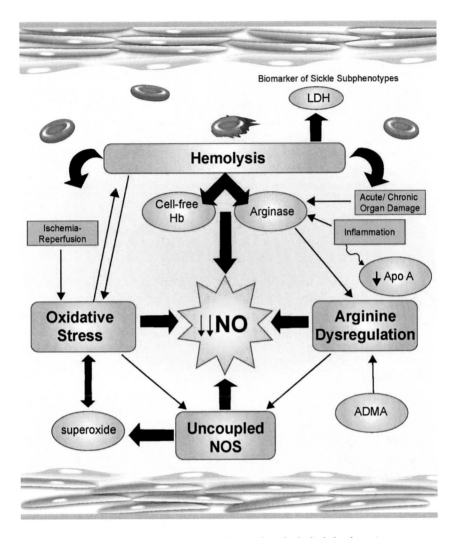

FIGURE 4-2 Mechanisms of vasculopathy and endothelial dysfunction.
NOTE: ADMA = asymmetric dimethylarginine; Apo A = apolipoprotein A-1; Hb = hemoglobin; LDH = lactate dehydrogenase; NO = nitric oxide; NOS = nitric oxide synthase.
SOURCES: As presented by Claudia Morris, April 2, 2018; Morris, 2008. Republished with permission of the American Society of Hematology. From Mechanisms of vasculopathy in sickle cell disease and thalassemia, Morris, C. R., 2008: 177–185. Permission conveyed through Copyright Clearance Center, Inc.

mentation with arginine, significant reduction in estimated pulmonary systolic pressures were seen, similar to the ones seen with medications. They identified a similar pattern of dysregulated arginine metabolism in patients with thalassemia, another hemolytic anemia associated with a high prevalence of pulmonary hypertension, but only in the group of patients at risk of pulmonary hypertension (Morris et al., 2005b). These data suggest a role for arginine bioavailability in the development of hemolysis-associated pulmonary hypertension. Surprisingly, low arginine bioavailability was associated with worse survival, and this was reflected by the arginine-to-ornithine ratio and also the global arginine bioavailability ratio. No deaths occurred in the patients who had the highest arginine bioavailability after 5 years of follow-up (Morris et al., 2005a).

Impact of a Disease State on Nutrient Metabolism and Nutritional Status

Arginine deficiency syndromes share similarities regardless of whether they mechanistically result from trauma, hepatic disease, an immune disorder, hemolyzed red cells during hemolysis or transfusion, or clinical consequences of excess extracellular arginase. In Morris's thinking, these syndromes fall into two baskets: endothelial dysfunction, which occurs in sickle cell disease as a model, and T-cell dysfunction, which is seen in trauma.

Arginine is essential for naïve T-cell activation. In trauma, T-cell proliferation is blunted, interferon-gamma and interleukin-2 production is inhibited, and T-lymphocyte-mediated cytotoxicity and memory response are nearly completely abolished when arginine is depleted, all of which increases the risk of infection. Providing arginine to the culture media restores T-cell function.

This has important implications for the 10 percent of trauma patients who develop wound infections, which are the leading cause of late organ failure. Enhanced wound healing has been seen with arginine-fortified formulas given after trauma and hemorrhagic shock. The greatest benefits of arginine supplementation appear to be in surgical patients. However, Morris noted that careful patient selection is critical because some evidence also suggests harm in sepsis and following acute myocardial infarction.

Morris concluded her talk by pointing out the paucity of evidence in children with sickle cell, particularly in terms of benefits associated with adequate protein intake. She also noted that it is important to remember that nutritional deficiencies rarely occur in isolation. Patients with sickle cell disease, for example, have a multitude of nutritional deficiencies that all must be addressed.

TRAUMATIC BRAIN INJURY: PATHOPHYSIOLOGICAL MECHANISMS AND POTENTIAL NUTRIENT NEEDS[2]

Both soldiers and civilians experience TBIs, but they are very different traumas. Military TBIs are mainly caused by blast traumatic injury, whereas civilians generally experience non-blast injuries caused by sports or motor vehicle accidents. About 87 percent of civilian TBI injuries, Scrimgeour said, are treated in emergency departments, and as many as 52,000 will die annually from a penetrating or severe TBI. Department of Defense (DoD) data from 2000 to 2017 indicate that nearly 380,000 service members were diagnosed with a TBI and about 82 percent of these injuries were classified as mild TBI. In the future, modern imaging techniques might allow the discrimination between mild TBIs that need treatment and those that will resolve on their own within a year. Despite DoD spending more than $940 million on TBI research, no pharmacological agents have been approved for soldiers exposed to TBI.

Scrimgeour noted that the 2011 Institute of Medicine (IOM) report *Nutrition and Traumatic Brain Injury* provides the foundation for existing thinking about nutritional support to improve acute and subacute health outcomes in military personnel who have experienced TBI (IOM, 2011). He then discussed the following recommendations from this report that are of particular relevance to the workshop:

- Recommendation 6-1 concerns the provision of early nutrition support, particularly protein. Scrimgeour noted that soldiers who have experienced a TBI often get little or no nutritional support, or interrupted nutritional support, during the immediate period after the blast injury, during the initial care in the combat hospital, and during the medical evacuation to Germany and eventually to Walter Reed National Military Medical Center in Bethesda, Maryland.
- Recommendations 5-1 and 5-2 urge DoD to conduct dietary intake assessments in military settings and on TBI patients in medical treatment facilities. Scrimgeour acknowledged that these assessments can be done in the United States, but they are much more difficult to do overseas.
- Recommendations 6-2 and 6-3 pertain to human trials to determine appropriate levels of blood glucose following TBI and of the appropriateness of insulin therapy in treating hyperglycemia observed in soldiers exposed to TBI in inpatient settings using total parenteral nutrition. Scrimgeour stated that his group has measured blood glucose in animal models with blast injuries compared to con-

---

[2] This section summarizes information presented by Angus Scrimgeour.

trols and found no change in blood glucose that would warrant intervention.

- Recommendation 9-1 concerns DoD monitoring the outcomes of a clinical trial on the effect of cytidine diphosphate (CDP)-choline on cognition and functional measures in severe, moderate, and complicated mild TBI. Scrimgeour stated that the 4-year trial was terminated early because of lack of results and that no further human trials have been conducted with CDP-choline.
- Recommendation 10-1 focused on studies to assess the use of creatine in TBI treatments, which has been shown to help sports athletes recover from muscle injury. Scrimgeour noted that no such human trials have been conducted and none are planned.
- Recommendation 13-1 states that DoD should conduct animal and human studies of omega-3 fatty acids. Scrimgeour noted that his lab is studying a docosahexaenoic acid–eicosapentaenoic acid (DHA-EPA) mix to determine whether it could help reduce neuro-inflammation in brains exposed to TBI, and minimize cognitive deficits. In addition, he said several double-blind randomized controlled trials are currently looking at the effects of a mix of DHA or DHA and EPA supplementation on concussion, and these trials will have results in the coming years.

Scrimgeour then reviewed the following nutritional recommendations from the IOM report and provided an update of work in those areas:

- **Zinc.** Evidence indicates that in a mildly zinc-deficient state animals do not recover after exposure to blast. To date, no human studies have been done since the 2011 report was published, although preclinical studies have shown that after an initial period of total parenteral nutrition, zinc supplementation increases visceral protein mass in post-TBI patients (Cope et al., 2012).
- **Curcumin.** Despite the data from animal studies showing benefits of curcumin supplementation following neurotrauma (Sharma et al., 2009, 2010; Zhu et al., 2014), no human trials have been conducted.
- **Resveratrol.** Two animal studies have shown some benefits with the use of resveratrol in concussion treatment (Lin et al., 2014; Singleton et al., 2010), and a double-blind study at The University of Texas Southwest Medical Center has looked at 500 milligrams of resveratrol in boxers. The Texas study has ended but has not been published.
- **Vitamin D.** Vitamin D has shown some promise for TBI in combination with progesterone in preliminary studies (Aminmansour

et al., 2012; Tang et al., 2013, 2015). However, the large phase III ProTECT (Progesterone for the Treatment of TBI) and SyNAPse (Efficacy and Safety Study of Progesterone in Patients with Severe TBI) trials were suspended due to lack of efficacy.

To summarize, Scrimgeour stated that evidence-based nutrition guidelines are lacking. Adequate, validated biomarkers for TBI are also lacking, making it difficult to identify targets for studies. To exacerbate the situation, Scrimgeour added, an overlap exists between TBI symptoms and posttraumatic stress disorder symptoms. Additionally, polytrauma is common in soldiers, and so it is not uncommon for physicians to provide treatment for shrapnel wounds, lacerations, or dizziness, but not the TBI due to a lack of neurotherapeutics.

METABOLIC TURNOVER, INFLAMMATION, AND REDISTRIBUTION: IMPACT ON NUTRIENT REQUIREMENTS[3]

Because of experiments with human study participants and animal models, it was previously thought that much was known about the requirements for vitamin B6 in humans. However, Gregory stated, that has changed considerably in recent years.

In most developed countries vitamin B6 status is generally adequate. The primary biomarker used in screening studies to assess B6 status, pyridoxal phosphate (PLP), is involved in more than 160 enzymatic reactions in the body, including amino acid metabolism, gluconeogenesis, and many one-carbon metabolism reactions. The current Recommended Dietary Allowance (RDA) for B6 is based on a cutoff of 20 nanomoles per liter of circulating PLP[4] (IOM, 1998). The most recent published National Health and Nutrition Examination Survey (NHANES) study that provided B6 data showed that only about 10 to 12 percent of the NHANES population of all of the different groups had less than the 20 nanomoles per liter (Pfeiffer et al., 2013).

Disease Relationships with Vitamin B6

Since the mid- to late 1990s, a number of published papers have shown a relationship between low plasma PLP and risk of vascular disease, which includes heart disease, risk of death from heart disease, stroke, and venous thrombosis (e.g., Rimm et al., 1998). Other studies also

---

[3] This section summarizes information presented by Jesse Gregory.
[4] See http://nationalacademies.org/HMD/Activities/Nutrition/SummaryDRIs/DRI-Tables.aspx (accessed June 6, 2018).

show an association between low PLP and C-reactive protein (CRP), an inflammatory marker, and disease severity in inflammatory bowel disease (IBD) and rheumatoid arthritis, both inflammatory diseases (Sakakeeny et al., 2012). The authors observed that PLP was inversely associated with many biomarkers of inflammation, not just CRP.

Gregory also described a study in which the apparent requirement for vitamin B6 was increased due to inflammatory disease itself, as reflected by CRP (Morris et al., 2010). One explanation is that PLP can be redistributed in the body from the more kinetically mobile pools to sites of inflammation. It has been shown that approximately 70 percent of vitamin B6 is tightly bound in muscle glycogen phosphorylase. However, the other 20 or 30 percent in liver and other organs is kinetically mobile and can be relocated to sites of inflammation as needed for metabolic demands in the inflammatory response. This has been demonstrated in a rat study, which showed liver and plasma PLP levels decreased as a result of an adjuvant injection, presumably to support the inflammation (Chiang et al., 2005). A second explanation is that some acceleration of B6 catabolism may occur during inflammation, as suggested by studies showing that the ratio of pyridoxic acid in plasma to its active forms, PLP and pyridoxal, is increased. It appears then that PLP has limitations as a biomarker when inflammatory conditions exist. Other biomarkers, such as erythrocyte transaminase stimulation assay, erythrocyte PLP, and urinary pyridoxic acid also have limitations. The most effective metabolic marker is plasma cystathionine, an intermediate in the trans-sulfuration pathway that takes homocysteine to cysteine and then glutathione. The kynurenines, which are in the tryptophan pathway, have been known for many years to be altered in B6 deficiency, and the ratio of hydroxyl-kynurenine to xanthurenic acid is a good biomarker that is little influenced by inflammation. However, these alternative biomarkers require further validation.

In summary, PLP is a very good biomarker for healthy people, but its responsiveness to inflammation raises questions about its value in assessing populations and in developing an RDA for B6, particularly because inflammation can be prevalent in the general population. The ratios of tryptophan catabolites do seem like an encouraging approach to developing a biomarker that is less sensitive to inflammation, but validation in terms of cutoffs, adequacy, and deficiency is needed.

MODERATED PANEL DISCUSSION AND Q&A

In response to a question related to L-arginine and wound healing, Morris replied that in adults, decreased mortality and morbidity are seen in some cohorts of patients who were fed arginine-fortified formulas. This is particularly true for surgical patients, although, she added, colleagues conducting these studies have found it difficult to convince surgeons to embrace this sort of nutritional intervention even when presented with rigorous evidence from clinical trials. Unfortunately, little data are available in children. Although it makes sense to think about therapeutics that involve arginase inhibitors, she said, given the critical roles of arginase in health, drugs that inhibit an enzyme that is so important must be pursued with great care.

Arginine and Glutamine

Morris replied to a question regarding FDA-approved glutamine. She noted that this is the first FDA-approved "drug" for children and only the second for adults with sickle cell disease but that its mechanism of action is still unknown. A number of pathways, including decreasing oxidative stress through NADPH (nicotinamide adenine dinucleotide phosphate), would make sense for sickle cell disease. Morris's thinking is that the glutamine is working through arginine, because glutamine is an arginine pro-drug. Arginine deficiency in sickle cell disease is associated with pulmonary hypertension, leg ulcers, and acute vaso-occlusive pain. These complications improve with arginine supplementation in clinical trials. She added that she has some pharmacokinetics data showing that a single dose of oral glutamine results in a significant increase in arginine bioavailability in patients with sickle cell disease. That suggests, she said, that glutamine does convert to arginine in sickle cell disease, which will ultimately improve arginine bioavailability both in plasma and within the red blood cell.

Responding to a question about the safety of arginine, Morris agreed there is reason for clinicians to be concerned because of the sepsis studies with arginine, but she emphasized that the nature of the patient population is important. Arginine is safe for sickle cell patients, most of whom are not septic but are arginine deficient. Sickle cell patients metabolize arginine differently than do normal controls, and arginine metabolism varies even in the same patient at steady-state compared to situations of acute illness including vaso-occlusive pain episodes. Ultimately, patients with sickle cell disease have a variable clinical spectrum of severity making treatment more complicated; sickle cell patients cannot all be treated in the same way.

Arginine and Trauma Recovery

To a question related to the use of omega-3 and arginine combinations that can get past the blood–brain barrier (BBB) and provide neuroprotective effects, Scrimgeour replied that his group has developed effective delivery systems to get omega-3 (specifically, DHA and EPA) and vitamin D into rats, with confirmation that these nutrients do cross the BBB. He also highlighted the distinction between non-blast TBI, common in sports and motor vehicle accidents, where the injury is restricted to the brain, and blast TBI, where the whole body is exposed, and intestinal damage frequently occurs.

Many soldiers also experience burn injuries. The animal models for burns are not optimal, and none of the current work conducted by the Army in San Antonio, Texas, is examining nutritional interventions. Zinc is leached out in the burn exudate, but studies on zinc supplements in burned animals and burned soldiers have not yet been conducted.

Limitations of Animal Models

On the limitations of animal models used to study TBI in soldiers, Scrimgeour responded that, contrary to humans with a rough (gyrencephalic) surface, the rat brain has a smooth (lissencephalic) surface and a different cortical bone thickness. He noted that multiple concerns exist about translating rat findings into humans, particularly in drug studies. For example, he said a Walter Reed lab has had very good success in drug studies repairing cognitive deficits as well as biochemical repair in the rat model, but it has not been possible to translate any of these findings into humans. It was noted that the same is true for IBD, in that animal models of IBD have terrible prognostic markers of therapeutics in human biology.

Using Technology to Understand Brain Biochemistry

The discussion highlighted that current technologies to understand how the brain is metabolically responding to a TBI, such as computed tomography scans, are not very sophisticated and that newer types of technology, such as 7T magnets used for functional magnetic resonance imaging and spectral imaging of the brain, could be applied. Although, currently, examinations of biomarkers of TBI can be done only after death, brain imaging technology and today's efforts in neuroscience may allow investigators to understand the human brain while people are still alive. In addition, there is the possibility of doing electroencephalography in the field for both athletes and soldiers.

REFERENCES

Aminmansour, B., H. Nikbakht, A. Ghorbani, M. Rezvani, P. Rahmani, M. Torkashvand, M. Nourian, and M. Moradi. 2012. Comparison of the administration of progesterone versus progesterone and vitamin D in improvement of outcomes in patients with traumatic brain injury: A randomized clinical trial with placebo group. *Advanced Biomedical Research* 1:58.

Chiang, E. P., D. E. Smith, J. Selhub, G. Dallal, Y. C. Wang, and R. Roubenoff. 2005. Inflammation causes tissue-specific depletion of vitamin B6. *Arthritis Research & Therapy* 7(6):R1254–R1262.

Cope, E. C., D. R. Morris, and C. W. Levenson. 2012. Improving treatments and outcomes: An emerging role for zinc in traumatic brain injury. *Nutrition Reviews* 70(7):410–413.

IOM (Institute of Medicine). 1998. *Dietary Reference Intakes for thiamin, riboflavin, niacin, vitamin B6, folate, vitamin B12, pantothenic acid, biotin, and choline.* Washington, DC: National Academy Press.

IOM. 2011. *Nutrition and traumatic brain injury: Improving acute and subacute health outcomes in military personnel.* Washington, DC: The National Academies Press.

Lin, C. J., T. H. Chen, L. Y. Yang, and C. M. Shih. 2014. Resveratrol protects astrocytes against traumatic brain injury through inhibiting apoptotic and autophagic cell death. *Cell Death & Disease* 5:e1147.

Morris, C. R. 2008. Mechanisms of vasculopathy in sickle cell disease and thalassemia. *Hematology American Society of Hematology Education Program* 177–185.

Morris, C. R., G. J. Kato, M. Poljakovic, X. Wang, W. C. Blackwelder, V. Sachdev, S. L. Hazen, E. P. Vichinsky, S. M. Morris, Jr., and M. T. Gladwin. 2005a. Dysregulated arginine metabolism, hemolysis-associated pulmonary hypertension, and mortality in sickle cell disease. *JAMA* 294(1):81–90.

Morris, C. R., F. A. Kuypers, G. J. Kato, L. Lavrisha, S. Larkin, T. Singer, and E. P. Vichinsky. 2005b. Hemolysis-associated pulmonary hypertension in thalassemia. *Annals of the New York Academy of Sciences* 1054:481–485.

Morris, M. S., L. Sakakeeny, P. F. Jacques, M. F. Picciano, and J. Selhub. 2010. Vitamin B-6 intake is inversely related to, and the requirement is affected by, inflammation status. *The Journal of Nutrition* 140(1):103–110.

Pfeiffer, C. M., M. R. Sternberg, R. L. Schleicher, B. M. Haynes, M. E. Rybak, and J. L. Pirkle. 2013. The CDC's *Second National Report on Biochemical Indicators of Diet and Nutrition in the U.S. Population* is a valuable tool for researchers and policy makers. *The Journal of Nutrition* 143(6):938S–947S.

Rimm, E. B., W. C. Willett, F. B. Hu, L. Sampson, G. A. Colditz, J. E. Manson, C. Hennekens, and M. J. Stampfer. 1998. Folate and vitamin B6 from diet and supplements in relation to risk of coronary heart disease among women. *JAMA* 279(5):359–364.

Sakakeeny, L., R. Roubenoff, M. Obin, J. D. Fontes, E. J. Benjamin, Y. Bujanover, P. F. Jacques, and J. Selhub. 2012. Plasma pyridoxal-5-phosphate is inversely associated with systemic markers of inflammation in a population of U.S. adults. *The Journal of Nutrition* 142(7):1280–1285.

Sharma, S., Y. Zhuang, Z. Ying, A. Wu, and F. Gomez-Pinilla. 2009. Dietary curcumin supplementation counteracts reduction in levels of molecules involved in energy homeostasis after brain trauma. *Neuroscience* 161(4):1037–1044.

Sharma, S., Z. Ying, and F. Gomez-Pinilla. 2010. A pyrazole curcumin derivative restores membrane homeostasis disrupted after brain trauma. *Experimental Neurology* 226(1):191–199.

Singleton, R. H., H. Q. Yan, W. Fellows-Mayle, and C. E. Dixon. 2010. Resveratrol attenuates behavioral impairments and reduces cortical and hippocampal loss in a rat controlled cortical impact model of traumatic brain injury. *Journal of Neurotrauma* 27(6):1091–1099.

Tang, H., F. Hua, J. Wang, I. Sayeed, X. Wang, Z. Chen, S. Yousuf, F. Atif, and D. G. Stein. 2013. Progesterone and vitamin D: Improvement after traumatic brain injury in middle-aged rats. *Hormones and Behavior* 64(3):527–538.

Tang, H., F. Hua, J. Wang, S. Yousuf, F. Atif, I. Sayeed, and D. G. Stein. 2015. Progesterone and vitamin D combination therapy modulates inflammatory response after traumatic brain injury. *Brain Injury* 1–10.

Zhu, H. T., C. Bian, J. C. Yuan, W. H. Chu, X. Xiang, F. Chen, C. S. Wang, H. Feng, and J. K. Lin. 2014. Curcumin attenuates acute inflammatory injury by inhibiting the TLR4/MyD88/NF-kappaB signaling pathway in experimental traumatic brain injury. *Journal of Neuroinflammation* 11:59.

5

Building the Evidence Base: Research Approaches for Nutrients in Disease States

Session 5 was moderated by Alex Kemper, Chief of the Division of Ambulatory Pediatrics at the Nationwide Children's Hospital and a member of the U.S. Preventive Services Task Force. The first presentation was delivered by Amanda MacFarlane, Research Scientist and Head of the Micronutrient Research Section in the Nutrition Research Division at Health Canada. MacFarlane discussed the type and strength of evidence needed to determine special nutrient requirements. The second talk, by Patrick Stover, Texas A&M AgriLife, focused on identifying and validating biomarkers in disease states. Nicholas Schork, Professor and Director of Human Biology at the J. Craig Venter Institute, delivered the next presentation, which examined innovative research designs aimed at determining efficacy of interventions. Two presentations then provided case examples of the issues involved in building an evidence base for special nutrient requirements for complex diseases. Gary Wu, Professor in Gastroenterology at the Perelman School of Medicine at the University of Pennsylvania and a Planning Committee member, discussed inflammatory bowel disease (IBD), and Steven Clinton, Professor in the Department of Internal Medicine at The Ohio State University and a Planning Committee member, discussed cancer. The session concluded with a moderated panel discussion and questions and answers with workshop participants.

TYPE AND STRENGTH OF EVIDENCE NEEDED FOR DETERMINING SPECIAL NUTRIENT REQUIREMENTS[1]

Dietary Reference Intake (DRI) values[2] are based on nutrient intakes and indicators, especially when talking about indicators of adequacy. The public health orientation of the DRIs, MacFarlane said, is that nutritional deficiencies in a population can be avoided. She added that the DRIs are also focused on adverse effects of high levels of intakes of specific nutrients (i.e., Tolerable Upper Intake Levels [ULs]). The DRIs are therefore based on data from apparently healthy populations and they apply to apparently healthy populations.

The DRIs do take into consideration the concept of chronic disease risk reduction, and, she clarified, that this has always been done when sufficient data for efficacy and safety exist. Additional guidance has recently been provided in the 2017 National Academies consensus study report *Guiding Principles for Developing Dietary Reference Intakes Based on Chronic Disease* (NASEM, 2017).

Adapting the Dietary Reference Intake Approach to Special Nutrient Requirements

MacFarlane continued, saying that the DRI approach has some fundamental aspects that could be adapted and potentially applied to special nutrient requirements and disease states. However, knowing that a relationship between nutrient and disease state exists is not sufficient to develop standards. To develop standards, she said, a certain level of evidence is needed. The first step in the risk assessment approach for setting DRIs is the demonstration of causality, which is the hazard identification (see Figure 5-1 and the presentation by Patsy Brannon in Chapter 1).

This requires a systematic review and, if possible, a meta-analysis of the literature. It also means interpretation of the data. As part of the systematic review, this process also includes the identification and selection of the appropriate indicators or endpoints, which, in the context of the DRIs, are health outcomes.

Once a causal relationship between the intake of a particular nutrient and a disease of deficiency is established, the next step is to model the intake–response relationship. The data required for this step are different from those required to identify a causal relationship. Data are needed to show, at multiple doses, that an association with the endpoint of inter-

---

[1] This section summarizes information presented by Amanda MacFarlane.

[2] For DRI values, see http://nationalacademies.org/HMD/Activities/Nutrition/Summary DRIs/DRI-Tables.aspx (accessed June 6, 2018).

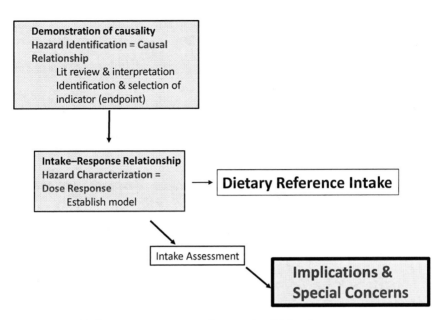

FIGURE 5-1 Risk assessment approach to setting DRI values.
SOURCE: As presented by Amanda MacFarlane, April 3, 2018.

est exists. Once that dose–response model is developed, it is possible to mathematically derive DRI values.

Finally, DRI committees do not end their work with setting the intake values. They also look at the intake assessment of the two populations of concern, which are Canada and the United States, to assess the risk of deficiency or excess. Additionally, DRI committees discuss implications and special concerns, for example, among specific population groups.

Applying the Dietary Reference Intake Risk Assessment Framework to Disease States

MacFarlane then turned her attention to applying this framework to nutrient requirements in specific disease states, arguing that some aspects of the DRI risk assessment approach are fundamental to establishing special nutrient requirement intake values in disease states.

Establishing Causality and Selecting Health Outcomes

When establishing causality, it is necessary to have a high level of confidence that an association exists between the exposure or intake of a given nutrient and the clinical outcome (see Figure 5-2). Therefore, identifying and selecting appropriate indicators of intake, status, and health outcome is critical.

Using the example of folate, in this figure, she said that folate intake modifies red blood cell folate (the indicator of status), which is directly linked to the clinical outcome, which is megaloblastic anemia. Vitamin C and scurvy and vitamin D and rickets are two other examples where a high level of certainty exists that the nutrient has a causal relationship with the endpoint of concern.

In the case of chronic disease, the aim is still to associate an exposure or intake with a clinical outcome, but the relationship is much more complicated. Essentially, a lower level of certainty of that relationship between the exposure and the clinical outcome or chronic disease exists, and it is often necessary to rely on the use of intermediate outcomes. MacFarlane then posed the question of how these relationships change when considering nutrient requirements for specific disease states. The direction of the relationship is different because instead of nutrient intake being associated with a disease of deficiency or chronic disease outcome, clinicians and investigators are looking at the disease state, which can affect exposure, and/or the indicator of status, and/or the clinical outcome associated with that indicator or status (see Figure 5-3). That is, the relationships are not always in one direction because the disease could have a direct impact on the outcome or vice versa, or because the disease itself could actually alter the biomarkers of status.

For example, IBD results in intestinal inflammation and malabsorption and is associated with low B vitamin and iron status and with anemia. The change in iron status could be the result of low iron intake or the result of the inflammation or malabsorption, that is, the disease itself. Another complicating factor in determining the outcome is the exposure.

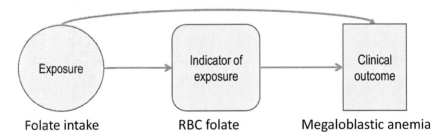

FIGURE 5-2 Establishing adequacy: Biomarkers of exposure on the causal pathway, using folate as an example.
NOTE: RBC = red blood cell.
SOURCE: As presented by Amanda MacFarlane, April 3, 2018.

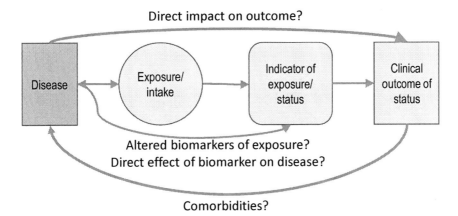

FIGURE 5-3 Nutrient requirements in disease states.
NOTES: The direction of the nutrient–disease relationship differs depending on which outcome is addressed by nutrient intake and whether it demonstrates an intake–response relationship. The further away from intake, the higher the potential is for uncertainty of relationships.
SOURCE: As presented by Amanda MacFarlane, April 3, 2018.

In the DRIs, the focus is dietary intake, but in disease states, the exposure could be intravenous, oral, or intraperitoneal. Every time the complexity increases, the level of uncertainty also increases. Cystic fibrosis (CF) is another good example of the complexities involved in establishing a special nutrient requirement for a disease (see Figure 5-4).

In this instance, the CF gene mutation is related to pancreatic insufficiency and to low status for fatty acids, fat soluble vitamins, proteins, and carbohydrates. All of these can be related to growth and bone health, with the latter being the traditional DRI health outcome associated with inadequate vitamin D. In this case, however, the CF presentation suggests that growth or lung function also could be the outcome of interest. It is critical to be transparent in these decisions, MacFarlane said, and to provide the data to support the decisions about selecting outcomes for establishing a special nutrient requirement for a disease.

Estimating Intake–Response Relationships

The next step is estimating intake–response relationships. For traditional diseases of deficiency, intakes are considered in terms of a threshold between what would be considered inadequate intakes and what would be considered safe and adequate. Traditionally, the gold standard for

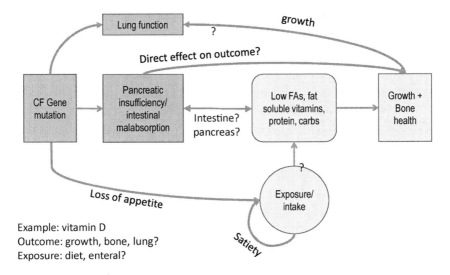

FIGURE 5-4 Example of complex relationships in cystic fibrosis.
NOTES: What could be selected as the outcome of interest when establishing the requirements for a nutrient such as vitamin D? This figure shows proof of principle in nature and does not represent the likely higher complexity of the nutrient–disease relationship. CF = cystic fibrosis; FA = fatty acid.
SOURCE: As presented by Amanda MacFarlane, April 3, 2018.

setting those thresholds is evidence from randomized controlled trials (RCTs) assessed through a systematic review and meta-analysis. Once those data have been obtained, it is possible to estimate the requirements. This becomes more difficult in the case of rare diseases, however, because evidence may be available on only a few people. Approaches to setting special nutrient requirements must consider the likelihood that a paucity of evidence exists. Future committees will have to grapple with questions about the acceptability of a lower level of evidence in the causal relationship and the ability to conduct dose–response modeling.

The Concept of Harm as It Applies to Dietary Reference Intakes

The DRIs focus not only on the low end of intakes but also include the UL, above which adverse effects may potentially occur. The DRIs also assume an interval of safe intakes between inadequacy and an UL. MacFarlane suggested that it could be argued that an interval of safe intakes may disappear when considering special nutrient requirements and disease states. Nutrient intakes in what would be considered the healthy range may actually pose harm for some, such as potassium in kidney disease, protein in phenylketonuria, or supplemental iron in hemochromatosis.

MacFarlane explained that it is even more complicated because the potential for overlap exists. For example, an increase in nutrient intake could decrease risk of one disease endpoint (or health outcome) but increase risk of another. For example, ketogenic diets for people with mitochondrial disease may have beneficial effects for patients with epilepsy, but they could also have dyslipidemic effects and thus exacerbate existing dyslipidemia.

Defining a Distinct Nutrient Requirement

MacFarlane then posed a basic question: How is "special" or "distinct" defined when talking about nutrient requirements? Is it simply a matter of a shift in the intake distribution? If it is just a matter of shifting the Estimated Average Requirement (EAR) to a lower level, for example, how different does the EAR have to be to be considered distinct? In the context of setting nutrient requirement values in disease states, the reality of making decisions may depend not only on differences in distribution of requirements but on other considerations as well, such as prevalence and severity of disease; disease activity (i.e., whether a person is in an active disease state or remission); presence of inflammation; effective dose, method of administration, and matrix (i.e., diet, supplement, formulated diet); sex and life stage; nutrient form (i.e., synthetic or natural); genetics of the individuals; confidence that everyone is equally responsive if extrapolation from one group to another is done; and maintenance of nutritional balance (i.e., whether the removal of one nutrient will adversely affect the nutritional balance of other nutrients).

In summary, MacFarlane said that aspects of the DRI risk assessment approach are applicable and adaptable to determining special nutrient requirements in disease states, but that any adaptation of the approach must be transparent. Moreover, decisions about defining the clinical population for such nutrient requirements and the level of evidence that will be used to set the requirements must be defined very carefully. In addition, clear and transparent analysis of the risks and benefits is needed, especially when they overlap. Rationales for extrapolation, if they are even acceptable, are needed, as are the inclusion and definition of any special considerations when setting special nutrient values.

IDENTIFICATION AND VALIDATION OF
BIOMARKERS IN DISEASE STATES[3]

Stover began his presentation by highlighting that when an individual has a chronic disease, the cutpoint between accumulated risk and actual disease onset is not well defined. In that way, the question becomes whether the disease trajectory can be measured, and how nutrition can modify that trajectory over the lifespan. The state of the art on knowledge of nutritional biomarkers has been covered in many excellent reports, Stover noted as he began his presentation. For example, the BOND (Biomarkers of Nutrition for Development) Program report defined "biomarker" as a distinct biological or biologically derived molecule found in blood or other bodily fluids or tissues that is a sign of a process, event, condition, or disease (Raiten et al., 2011). Stover explained that measuring nutrient-specific biomarkers can determine exposure, identify changes in nutrient status, clarify function within the body, and indicate direct and indirect effects on systems.

When classifying and evaluating human nutrient needs in disease states, it is desirable to have a good indicator or biomarker of the disease itself and its severity. In addition, it is desirable to have measures that indicate whole body nutritional status, biomarkers for normal physiological function and clinical outcomes, and predictive biomarkers in terms of future chronic disease risk that may even be independent of the current disease state. In considering these measures, Stover noted that comorbidities must also be considered.

Evaluation of Biomarkers and Surrogate Endpoints in Chronic Disease, a report on the current state of evaluation of biomarkers and surrogate endpoints in chronic disease, discusses validated surrogate biomarkers, that is, biomarkers that directly relate a nutrient intake to a health outcome along a causal pathway (IOM, 2010). Because validated surrogate biomarkers are not common, non-validated intermediate functional biomarkers are often used, explained Stover. These biomarkers may not necessarily relate to a clinical outcome but indicate a dose–response relationship between a nutrient intake level and a physiological response.

The challenge in thinking about chronic disease, stated Stover, is that it can often be tissue specific. As a result, measuring the systemic nutrient status might not be appropriate. A good example, Stover noted, is the blood–brain barrier (BBB), where it may not be possible to detect what may be occurring in the brain if some disease process is occurring in brain tissue only. Functional biomarkers can provide insights into the physiology and pathology of a specific tissue.

---

[3] This section summarizes information presented by Patrick Stover.

In the case of disease, Stover noted that it is important to determine what is being measured—the whole body, tissue, or the cell. Moreover, the major interest for biomarkers is in disease progression and/or comorbidities related to the disease-induced nutritional deficiency. For example, if certain proteins that are present in cerebrospinal fluid, such as s100beta and glial fibrillary acidic protein (GFAP), appear in the blood, this would potentially be an indication of a dysfunctional BBB, which could be used as a proxy for nutrient deficiencies in the brain. This type of biomarker could help in predicting nutrient deficiencies in certain diseases.

Precision Medicine

Predictive biomarkers are needed that can help clarify what nutrients will be affected by a disease, and whether increased input of that nutrient will affect a deficiency. Once those questions are answered, then other nutritional biomarkers can be used to determine the dose–response relationship that is required to meet that new requirement in the disease.

Stover noted that one of the challenges, however, is that as a disease progresses in severity, nutrient needs are altered. However, new, inexpensive, microfluidic devices (the same technologies used for pregnancy tests) are being developed that can yield immediate real-time readouts of nutritional and disease status, allowing individuals to make real-time adjustments. Many companies are commercializing these point-of-care diagnostics, said Stover, showing that technology may be ahead of current science.

Disease Modifies Nutrition Status and Nutritional Biomarkers

Complex relationships sometimes exist between disease and biomarkers. For example, the BRINDA (Biomarkers Reflecting Inflammation and Nutritional Determinants of Anemia) project (https://brinda-nutrition. org), which seeks to examine the relationship between inflammation and biomarkers, contends that acute and chronic inflammation can modify nutrient biomarker measures and inflammation can have a direct effect on actual nutrient status. To support these points, BRINDA investigators concluded that the prevalence of low total body iron is underestimated if it is not adjusted for inflammation (Mei et al., 2017). That means, said Stover, that biomarkers in a disease state must be adjusted in order to fully understand actual nutritional status.

In conclusion, Stover pointed to the need for systems biomarkers. These are needed in part because many of the specific tissues of interest are not accessible for measurement. To illustrate, Stover described ongoing work by Karsten Hiller in Germany, who is investigating whether people with diabetes can be classified in terms of their Cori cycle functionality, which could in turn serve as a biomarker to prescribe either nutrients, diet, or drugs to treat that diabetes. Hiller and his team are now examining the potential for dietary interventions to see how diet can modify the Cori cycle in various disease states.

INNOVATIVE CAUSAL DESIGNS FOR EFFICACY: WHAT TYPE OF EVIDENCE IS NEEDED?[4]

New legislation, such as the 21st Century Cures Act, will have substantial implications for how evidence is brought to the U.S. Food and Drug Administration (FDA). The 21st Century Cures Act, explained Schork, calls for a reconsideration of the RCT, and perhaps even the substitution of RCTs with data summaries and real-world evidence. FDA has released a number of reports that advocate for these changes, including the idea to substitute Phase III and Phase IV clinical trials with "learning systems." These systems provide a way to collect data on people, through approaches such as mining electronic medical records to look for trends that might be clinically useful for patients in the future.

N-of-1 Trials

Schork then described N-of-1 trials, a good example of the trend toward real-world evidence that has been gaining attention in recent years. In N-of-1 trials, a clinician takes a baseline measure, then provides an intervention to the patient and records clinical measures. The clinician may decide at some point to stop that intervention and try an alternative. The intervention(s) are done some number of times, with the clinician recording the clinical measure throughout the cycle of alternating treatments. This focus on helping a patient get better, rather than solely on evaluating an intervention, allows clinicians to test multiple interventions, and so long as the condition is not acute and life threatening, the clinician can see which one performs optimally for the patient. It is possible to provide this trial to multiple patients, where one patient may respond to one intervention, and another may respond to a different intervention. Data can be collected on these individuals to enable claims about correlations between the changes in the clinical parameter and certain measures. These trials leverage big data for individual patients to allow conclusions about health status in response to many kinds of interventions.

---

[4] This section summarizes information presented by Nicholas Schork.

Many of the initial N-of-1 trials were not done with a great deal of rigor and guides on conducting these studies have since been published. Schork emphasized that the power of N-of-1 studies is not due to the number of participants. It is due to the number of observations that can be made and the study designs that are used to make causal claims about the influence of an intervention on a clinically meaningful parameter. This approach is fundamentally different than the way historical population-based trials have been pursued.

Schork illustrated the methodology of N-of-1 trials by showing several different study designs. For example, a sequential nature design could be used if the clinician wants to minimize the amount of time that a patient is on one therapy because evidence is building that another therapy is more beneficial. Trial designs can also be optimized to minimize the amount of time a patient is on a less beneficial trial but still allow enough data to be collected to make objective claims about the efficacy of a particular intervention. For example, if a clinician is contrasting two interventions and wants to optimize the distribution of a finite number of measurements, one way to optimize the design of having the patient be on alternating treatments is to rotate the number of times the patient is on each intervention. In this way, the data that are generated are not influenced by the overt serial correlation between the observations. Collecting data on a single individual will result in strong correlations between the measures and with an assumption about the strength of the serial correlation, it is possible to optimize these designs to maximize the power to bring out one effect over another.

Explaining further, Schork said that it is also possible to aggregate N-of-1 studies into clusters and identify trends and factors in common (e.g., a genotype or a specific environmental exposure) to predict the best intervention for future patients.

Personal Versus Population Thresholds

Schork continued with another aspect of N-of-1 trials, which illustrates personal versus population thresholds. He used the example of a clinician with cholesterol measures on 25 individuals. Some of these individuals may have a cholesterol number that is greater than the population threshold (e.g., 200 mg/mL).

If one of those individuals has fairly low cholesterol values, a personal average for that patient could be established and perhaps errors could also be established. Over time, it could be observed that the patient's cholesterol level has deviated significantly from his initial values but is still below the population threshold. The increased trend, however, might indicate a health status change, despite the fact that the cholesterol level is below the population threshold. This idea has been used to illustrate the identification of ovarian cancer about 1 year before population thresholds would have indicated the disease (Speake et al., 2017).

Identifying, Verifying, and Vetting Nutrition Strategies for Individuals

The use of vetting algorithms to match nutritional interventions to patient profiles is also gaining ground, Schork said. This approach uses an entire battery of omics profiling to determine what kind of perturbations might be present in any one individual's profile; the results can be used to identify an optimal diet or supplementation intervention.

In this approach, it is important to identify a strategy for matching the profiles to the nutritional interventions, recognizing that what is actually being tested is an algorithm, not an individual intervention. To illustrate, Schork noted that individual cancer patients' tumors exhibit perturbations and certain drugs can uniquely counteract the pathophysiology induced by those specific tumor mutations. To identify matches between tumor perturbations that might be unique to a small set of the population and specific drugs, cancer clinicians would have to run many trials with small numbers of patients, and that would be inefficient. The cancer community has developed an alternative strategy, called "bucket" or "basket" or "umbrella" trials, in which a treatment basket is given to an individual based on the perturbations profile of the tumor. It is not the individual drugs, but the perturbations that are being tested, a crucial difference in the approach to vetting interventions.

Schork then reviewed the following questions raised by this approach:

- What happens if the trial fails? For example, in a recent basket trial, patients experienced no better outcomes than people that received the standard of care. Although these results generated considerable concern about the approach of personalized oncology, a key message was that the community must look critically at the basis for the matching algorithm before discarding the whole field of personalized oncology or personalized nutrition.
- How should insights that arise external to the trial be accommodated? For example, what happens if the day after a basket trial begins, *Nature* publishes a paper saying people with the HER2 perturbation should get a different drug than the one prescribed in the trial? The solution may be to allow the trial rules to be adapted over time, even though that solution would be difficult for the biostatisticians analyzing the data.

Other issues to consider relate to whether the perturbations in the tumor can be assessed properly, the nature of the algorithm itself, and the role of the Tumor Board, which decides whether oncology drugs that were recommended by the algorithm are likely to benefit the patient. Similar issues could occur if algorithms were used to guide nutrition interventions. Schork concluded his presentation by noting that these issues raise the question of whether all the algorithms that are being developed by different groups should be vetted in a regulated environment.

EXAMPLES OF A COMPLEX DISEASE: INFLAMMATORY BOWEL DISEASE[5]

In wet bench research that uses animal model systems, animals have defined environmental conditions and genetics and a monotonous diet. Results from studies with these animals have a high signal-to-noise ratio, and it is possible to demonstrate proof of concept cause-and-effect relationships with a modest-sized cohort. In contrast, Wu explained, humans are free-living in a highly variable environment, with genetic diversity and a variable diet. As a result, this inter-subject variability results in a very low signal-to-noise ratio in many of the topics studied, making research in humans immensely complicated.

Given this reality, Wu said, an increasingly desired approach is to embrace the complexity of human biology through the use of high dimensional analytic technologies together with advanced computational biostatistical platforms. When doing human research, the goal is to match a physiological response with many different biospecimens, then run the data through very high throughput analytic technologies. Enormous databases are then generated that can be analyzed using the best medical approaches, bioinformatics, biostatistics, and computational biology to understand patterns and to identify and characterize biological mechanisms that drive the human response to an intervention.

The Example of Inflammatory Bowel Disease

The prevalence of IBD is high in the United States and worldwide. The genetic contribution to the development of Crohn's disease is at most 30 to 40 percent, and about 10 percent for ulcerative colitis. Environmental factors, including industrialization, are the largest contributor to the pathogenesis of IBD. Consideration, therefore, could be given to engineer the environment of the gut through diet, through the microbiome, or perhaps both to improve the efficacy of current therapeutic strategies focused on

---

[5] This section summarizes information presented by Gary Wu.

host immunosuppression. The gut microbiota is deeply dysbiotic in IBD, as the microbial community is responding to an environmental stress (i.e., inflammation of the intestinal tract). It is thought that this dysbiosis plays a role in perpetuating IBD. As a result, strategies have been developed to change the environment of the gut to alter dysbiosis in ways that favor the health of the host.

Dietary Intervention in Inflammatory Bowel Disease

Current treatments for Crohn's disease, such as metronidazole and ciprofloxacin, and fecal microbiota transplantation, do not work as robustly and as consistently as desired. This provides an opportunity to use the best technologies in human subject research to examine how altering the environment of the gut, perhaps through dietary interventions, might be beneficial in treating IBD. The paradigm being used to support this notion, said Wu, is that diet is epidemiologically associated with IBD, gut microbiota unquestionably play a role in the pathogenesis of IBD, and diet can shape the composition of the microbiota, which leads to the production of many different types of metabolites.

With this paradigm in mind, researchers have examined whether understanding the biological principles by which a specific diet is beneficial would inform efforts to design better diets for patients with IBD (see Figure 5-5). For example, defined formula diets for the treatment of Crohn's disease are most effective when they are consumed entirely in place of a normal diet (i.e., exclusive enteral nutrition [EEN]). This raises the question, explained Wu, of whether EEN provides something good, or excludes something bad, for patients with IBD that is different from the regular whole food diet. To understand EEN diets and their impact on IBD, investigators can study the microbiome by using DNA sequencing technologies or by identifying the metabolites that are made by these microbes because they may have an impact on the host.

Wu then described the Food and Resulting Microbial Metabolites (FARMM) study (part of the Crohn's & Colitis Foundation's Microbiome Initiative[6]), which explored the relationship between dietary composition, gut microbiome composition, and the metabolic products that are ultimately present in the gut lumen and in the plasma of humans. Healthy vegans and omnivores were randomized to consume an EEN diet. In the first period of the study, the researchers looked at the impact of these diets on the gut microbiome composition. Halfway through the intervention, the subjects' guts were purged, reducing bacterial load very substantially.

---

[6] See http://www.crohnscolitisfoundation.org/science-and-professionals/research/current-research-studies/microbiome-initiative.html (accessed June 14, 2018).

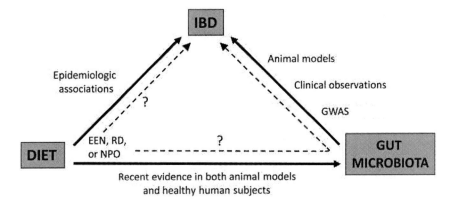

FIGURE 5-5 The relationship among diet, the gut microbiota, and IBD.
NOTE: EEN = exclusive enteral nutrition; GWAS = genome-wide association study; IBD = inflammatory bowel disease; NPO = nil per os (i.e., complete bowel rest); RD = restriction diet.
SOURCES: As presented by Gary Wu, April 3, 2018; Albenberg et al., 2012. Reprinted with permission from Wolters Kluwer: Albenberg, L. G., J. D. Lewis, and G. D. Wu. 2012. Food and the gut microbiota in inflammatory bowel diseases: A critical connection. *Current Opinion in Gastroenterology* 28(4):314–320. https:// journals.lww.com/co-gastroenterology/pages/default.aspx (accessed June 14, 2018).

Comparing the two time points would reveal differences in metabolites produced and consumed by microbes. As the microbiota reconstituted itself, the researchers could then correlate increases or decreases in metabolites with the occurrence of microbes and diet to identify key drivers.

Throughout the study, the team completed shotgun metagenomic sequencing of all the different stool samples. The team performed fecal and plasma metabolomics as well as collected rectal biopsies to isolate lamina propria mononuclear cells for analysis by a mass cytometry platform to understand how the mucosal immune system was actually responding at each of the different study intervals.

Wu then presented results showing numbers of different types of microbes in the gut environment based on the three different diets. The vegan microbiome was more resilient to environmental stress than the omnivore microbiome based on the ability of the gut microbiome to reconstitute itself after flushing of the gut. The gut microbiota of study participants on an EEN diet was the least resilient. Wu also presented data using a novel statistical approach suggesting that EEN excludes some metabolites that are in whole food diets (some that plausibly could be bad for patients with IBD) as well as includes other metabolites provided by EEN that may not be present in whole food diets (some that plausibly could be beneficial for patients with IBD).

In a second study of diet, the plasma metabolome, and the microbiota of vegans and omnivores, a heat map of different nutrients in diets showed, not surprisingly, substantial differences between the vegans and the omnivores. Results from the plasma metabolome showed a similar result. A random forest algorithm, a machine learning tool that helps identify features that determine a dichotomous outcome, was able to predict with 94 percent accuracy whether an individual was a vegan or an omnivore, simply by looking at 30 small molecules in blood, only 5 of which are generated by the gut microbiota. These results suggest that the main impact of diet on the human plasma metabolome is a direct effect on the host with a smaller contribution working through the gut microbiota.

EXAMPLES OF A COMPLEX DISEASE: CANCER[7]

The World Cancer Research Fund and the American Institute for Cancer Research (WCRF-AICR) reports are the most authoritative global report on food, nutrition, nutrients, weight control, and physical activity.

Clinton stated that WCRF-AICR reports were published in 1997 and 2007 (WCRF-AICR, 1997, 2007). Since then, WCRF-AICR has conducted a continuous update program to review the data for three or four cancers per year. All of these will be compiled into a new report that will be published in 2018. An international panel of 20 to 25 leaders in the field and more that 250 reviewers and contributors around the world participated in its development, which was based on systematic reviews and meta-analyses. Clinton summarized the WCRF-AICR nutrition-related recommendations as the following:

- **Body fatness:** Be as lean as possible within the normal range of body weight.
- **Foods and drinks that promote weight gain:** Limit consumption of energy-dense foods. Avoid sugary drinks.
- **Plant foods:** Eat mostly foods of plant origin.
- **Animal foods:** Limit intake of red meat and avoid processed meat.
- **Alcoholic drinks:** Limit alcoholic drinks.
- **Preservation, processing, preparation:** Limit consumption of salt. Avoid moldy grains or legumes.
- **Dietary supplements:** Aim to meet nutritional needs through diet alone.

---

[7] This section summarizes information presented by Steven Clinton.

The WCRF-AICR reports make no specific nutrient requirement recommendations, such as DRIs related to cancer outcomes, because the data have not reached a sufficient level of scientific rigor to make such recommendations. The WCRF-AICR strength of the evidence for recommendations are categorized as convincing, probable, limited but suggestive, or a substantial effect is unlikely.

The *Dietary Guidelines for Americans* policy document, which was based in large part on an expert committee's technical report, also makes no specific nutrient requirement recommendations regarding cancer. Rather, the focus of the 2015–2020 *Dietary Guidelines for Americans* was dietary patterns. Overall, the dietary patterns recommended in the *Dietary Guidelines for Americans* are consistent with the WCRF-AICR recommendations.

Effect of Nutrients on the Cancer Continuum

Clinton then addressed how different phases of the cancer continuum have implications for nutrition and nutrient requirements. For example, all of the factors that enhance cancer risk will require unique and specific nutritional interventions; cancer treatment has numerous nutrition-related impacts; and the end-of-life phase has significant nutrition implications, including malnutrition related to pain management, cachexia, and sarcopenia. Nutrition is also a critical issue for the millions of cancer survivors, as cancer therapies increase the risk of obesity, metabolic syndrome, and fitness issues. Hearing, taste, neuropathies, gastrointestinal dysfunction, cardiopulmonary disease, long-term heart function, and reproductive and renal issues are all prevalent based on different cancer therapies. Clinton stated that nutritional interventions clearly may play a role in many of these processes.

The Complexity of Host Genetics

Clinton then briefly discussed how host genetics affect many aspects of cancer biology within an individual. These include the more than 50 inherited cancer syndromes and cancer susceptibility genes, such as BRCA1 for breast cancer, adenomatous polyposis coli (APC) for polyposis coli, retinal blastoma, and p53 for Li-Fraumeni syndrome. Many of these mutations are of low prevalence and contribute to only a small proportion of the human cancer burden.

In contrast, host susceptibility genes, such as polymorphisms and variations in cytochrome p450s, have high prevalence. The absolute risk associated with any one of these genes is low, but the attributed risk can be much higher. One example is p53, the gene related to Li-Fraumeni syndrome, which can lead to sarcomas and breast, leukemia, lung, brain, and adrenal cancers.

Clinton then explained that murine models and very simple studies in mice have demonstrated that nutritional status can alter the biology of inherited cancer syndromes. For example, a 1994 study looking at caloric restriction and spontaneous tumorigenesis in the p53 knockout mice found a fairly strong inhibitory effect of calorie restriction on the development of this disease in the murine models (Hursting et al., 1994). Translating to a human system, Clinton noted that similar results could easily mean 20 to 30 years of added life for an individual with Li-Fraumeni syndrome. Clinton concluded that dozens of nutrients may affect the cancer process and human studies are desperately needed to define DRIs that may be relevant to inherited cancer syndromes.

The Complexity of Cancer Genetics

Moving on to the genetics of cancer itself, Clinton said that this is where the real complexity lies. This is illustrated by the National Institutes of Health's Cancer Genome *Pan-Cancer Atlas* (https://cancergenome.nih.gov), a national effort to define the landscape of the mutational signatures across human cancers, through integrating omics across platforms from human samples.

Even though the mutational landscape is large, the array of driver mutations is more limited. These mutations drive certain critical biological processes, such as evading growth suppression, avoiding immune recognition and destruction, tumor-associated inflammation, and angiogenesis. Addressing these "hallmarks of cancer" is key to successful treatment. Cancer evolves with more and different mutations as it goes through the therapeutic and metastatic process, and although driver mutations may be present in the early stages up through diagnosis, treatment may eliminate certain clones and allow others to grow and progress. Achieving cures in such types of malignancy where different metastatic sites with very different mutational patterns exist in a single individual is very difficult.

Special Nutrient Requirements in Cancer

Clinton concluded his presentation with the following comments about DRIs and cancer:

- Developing DRIs for cancer prevention using the public health approach should and will continue.

- The complexity of cancer and the unique aspect of each individual's experience will drive efforts toward personalized nutrition therapy. New study designs, such as N-of-1 trials and personalized treatment, are very relevant to the food and nutrition aspects of cancer.
- Improved technology permits a more precise definition of nutritional status in each individual in real time, and this will allow for more efficient, effective, and meaningful applications to each person. Much more research is needed to define efficacy and safety of interventions.
- Currently, most cancer patients do not have optimal access to nutrition support services. This requires changes in reimbursement and full integration of the expertise from registered dietitians (RDs) into programs at hospitals. RD researchers are desperately needed to do the science to define future interventions.
- A category of bioactive food components should be formally established to encompass components such as fiber and polyphenols. The term *nutrient* should be limited to those compounds that have a defined deficiency syndrome that is immediately reversed by replacing that component. Efforts should be pursued to define optimal intake of these bioactive food components.

MODERATED PANEL DISCUSSION AND Q&A

As the presenters gathered for the panel discussion, Kemper reflected on the theme of tension, which emerged across the presentations. This included the tension of the single nutrient versus the dietary pattern, the tension of genes versus the environment, the tension between understanding things at the population level versus personalized medicine, the tension of traditional RCTs versus N-of-1 study designs, and the tension between looking at final health outcomes versus intermediate biomarkers.

Patient Perspectives on Developing Nutrient Recommendations

To a question related to the patient perspective in establishing nutrient requirements and the feasibility of individuals changing their diet, MacFarlane responded that a regulatory body's responsibility would be to have good standards based on good evidence of what disease responds to what particular nutrient intake. Other groups with other responsibilities, such as health care providers, the food industry, and the insurance industry would also need to be involved.

Dietary Recommendations When Good Biomarkers Are Not Available

A discussion was initiated on the question of how to pursue research when a paucity of good biomarkers for some diseases, such as irritable bowel syndrome or even osteoarthritis exists. Wu responded by suggesting that biomarkers might not be available because researchers have not looked hard enough. For example, a somewhat controversial dietary intervention for the treatment of IBD is a low fermentable oligosaccharides, disaccharides, monosaccharides, and polyols (FODMAP) diet. If one were to ask what happens to the metabolome on the low FODMAP diet, and the diet is matched to bacterial taxa, or one asks what happens to the metabolome of plasma and the feces, it might be possible to identify biomarkers that might actually predict somebody's response to the low FODMAP diet.

Schork added that to discover such biomarkers, better designs to get at causal relationships between, for example, variables that are measured routinely on individuals and outcomes of relevance might be needed. For example, very large observational studies are valuable, but this design is not able to separate the findings that might be secondary to the intervention being used.

Wu then added that researchers have increasingly begun to conduct association studies using omic technologies. Even though the reasons for the association may not be clear, these studies are enormously valuable because if a wet bench researcher can phenocopy the association in a culture system and/or in an animal model, it might help show more about cause-and-effect relationships that drive the biological process in human biology.

What Level of Evidence Is Necessary?

Wu then followed up this comment with a question for MacFarlane about the necessary level of evidence. If a study shows a very strong association between certain biomarkers and a certain outcome, would some type of cause-and-effect evidence still be necessary? If a laboratory were able to provide very strong evidence of a biological process in an animal model, must it also be proved in humans, or is the animal evidence a sufficient level of evidence? MacFarlane said that validation in humans still must be done. Animal models are critical for looking into the mechanisms underlying the associations being seen. Without validation in humans, however, the modeling would include a level of uncertainty that might not be acceptable.

Stover added to the discussion by saying that researchers would want to make sure, obviously, that a cause-and-effect relationship exists. He noted that the prevention of neural tube defects with folic acid comes to mind as an example. The reason why folic acid prevents neural tube defects is still unknown, but early clinical observations showed that at a certain level of exposure, 70 percent of these defects can be prevented. That level of exposure then became the standard of care. The World Health Organization (WHO) had to respond to countries who wanted to know how much folic acid should be put in the food supply. WHO used a big data approach, where they used observational data and big datasets to create a computed dose–response curve. The fortification amount was completely computed from observational data and then it was validated from very small clinical studies. However, no biomarkers that relate the exposure to the disease exist. In the ensuing discussion, MacFarlane responded that a causal effect was still demonstrated in an intervention trial first. A workshop participant added that decisions on folic acid fortification made by the FDA Folic Acid Subcommittee of the Food Advisory Committee were challenging because of the variability on dose response and level of toxicity, even though it was clear that a dose response existed. Clinton joined the conversation by pointing out that in some situations the rules can be bent; for example, public health recommendations around tobacco use in the 1960s were never based on an RCT of cigarette smoking and lung cancer because the evidence from observational studies was so strong. A comment was made that in contrast to the case of tobacco, in nutritional studies, the relative risks are almost invariably less than two and given the noise of food intake assessments, variability in composition of diets, and other unaccounted for variables in the environment, it is difficult to know when the signals are greater than the noise.

Bridging the Gap Between Evidence and Clinical Practice

A question was brought up related to the reluctance of some gastroenterologists to accept the contribution of diet to IBD when substantial evidence is accumulating in actual clinic practice. Wu added that the most frequent questions gastroenterologists hear from patients with IBD are related to diet. Although evidence exists, studies are often anecdotal or not well controlled or rigorous. Wu said that he thinks the defined formula diets probably reflect the best currently available evidence. Gastroenterologists and scientists have finally accepted the fact that diet does have an impact and if more funding becomes available, the field will be able to make progress and provide evidence-based recommendations about diet. He added that the only current evidence-based recommendation is that patients with Crohn's disease who may have intestinal strictures should avoid fibrous food products because it might lead to intestinal obstruction. Wu responded to a question related to noncompliance in following diets and implications for the specificity and sensitivity of the measurements with these metabolomic differences. Wu said that he attempts to control as many variables as possible so as to reduce the noise level and still see associations with a biomarker, which is then used in outpatient studies in a much larger group. A useful study to validate results would be to take various types of biomarkers that are seen in an inpatient setting, track them in an outpatient setting, and then ask several hundred individuals to complete a food frequency questionnaire or a dietary recall. This approach would allow researchers to assess methods that are currently considered to be the best way to understand what people are actually eating.

RCTs and N-of-1 Trials in an Era of Big Data

A comment was made related to increasing the power of N-of-1 studies by aggregating and using the results toward personalized nutrition categories over time. Schork replied that the NIH-funded Clinical and Translation Science Awards Program is pursuing efforts in this regard, for example, in having the nodes in the network interact to collect and share data. For many conditions, he said, the data to make good clinical decisions are insufficient, but an RCT in some cases may not be the best design to use to determine a better clinical course. One idea is to collect records on patients that could be predictive of a particular outcome and publish the results after a peer review process. On this basis, trends could be identified to help make decisions about optimal treatments. In the current era of big data, this approach would be feasible. A concern with the N-of-1 studies would be that an investigator justifies something post hoc. The idea of using algorithms has been challenged on the grounds that the fact that many studies might be consistent with a particular algorithm does not necessarily reveal causality. Schork agreed with this point, but also commented that RCTs rarely collect enough data on any one participant to say unequivocally whether that person responded to the treatment or not. The N-of-1 study designs are intended to bring out the response phenotype in ways that are more compelling than is possible in standard RCTs. In this era of personalized medicine and nutrition, the objective, Schork said, is to identify the responders and non-responders. Marriott added the final comment of the discussion session by noting that many states are now collecting very large datasets of individual data across hospitals, but protection of the data is essential for the public to be confident that their own personalized information will not be jeopardized.

REFERENCES

Albenberg, L. G., J. D. Lewis, and G. D. Wu. 2012. Food and the gut microbiota in inflammatory bowel diseases: A critical connection. *Current Opinion in Gastroenterology* 28(4):314–320.

Hursting, S. D., S. N. Perkins, and J. M. Phang. 1994. Calorie restriction delays spontaneous tumorigenesis in p53-knockout transgenic mice. *Proceedings of the National Academy of Sciences of the United States of America* 91(15):7036–7040.

IOM (Institute of Medicine). 2010. *Evaluation of biomarkers and surrogate endpoints in chronic disease.* Washington, DC: The National Academies Press.

Mei, Z., S. M. Namaste, M. Serdula, P. S. Suchdev, F. Rohner, R. Flores-Ayala, O. Y. Addo, and D. J. Raiten. 2017. Adjusting total body iron for inflammation: Biomarkers Reflecting Inflammation and Nutritional Determinants of Anemia (BRINDA) project. *The American Journal of Clinical Nutrition* 106(Suppl. 1):383S–389S.

NASEM (National Academies of Sciences, Engineering, and Medicine). 2017. *Guiding principles for developing Dietary Reference Intakes based on chronic disease.* Washington, DC: The National Academies Press.

Raiten, D. J., S. Namaste, B. Brabin, G. Combs, Jr., M. R. L'Abbe, E. Wasantwisut, and I. Darnton-Hill. 2011. Executive summary—Biomarkers of nutrition for development: Building a consensus. *The American Journal of Clinical Nutrition* 94(2):633S–650S.

Speake, C., E. Whalen, V. H. Gersuk, D. Chaussabel, J. M. Odegard, and C. J. Greenbaum. 2017. Longitudinal monitoring of gene expression in ultra-low-volume blood samples self-collected at home. *Clinical and Experimental Immunology* 188(2):226–233.

WCRF-AICR (World Cancer Research Fund and American Institute for Cancer Research). 1997. *Food, nutrition and the prevention of cancer: A global perspective.* Washington, DC: American Institute for Cancer Research.

WCRF-AICR. 2007. *Food, nutrition, physical activity, and the prevention of cancer: A global perspective.* Washington, DC: American Institute for Cancer Research.

6

Exploring Potential Opportunities

Session 6 was moderated by Barbara Schneeman, Professor Emerita at the University of California, Davis, and chair of the Planning Committee. The session opened with a panel that provided perspectives on the workshop's presentations from a variety of aspects. These presentations were followed by an open discussion and questions and answers with workshop participants. The session concluded with brief remarks by a speaker from each of the workshop sponsors. These speakers thanked the Planning Committee, presenters, and participants for a stimulating and thoughtful workshop and highlighted themes that complement their own organization's mission and initiatives.

Before introducing the first panel, Schneeman briefly summarized a few of the key themes that stood out to her over the course of the presentations and discussions. One theme that repeatedly emerged was the importance of understanding the difference between approaches for treating, curing, or preventing disease, and approaches for managing a disease so that the person's health improves by compensating for what the disease is doing to nutrient metabolism. Sometimes a drug is involved with managing disease, but sometimes the management issues are related to different nutrient requirements. Another theme for Schneeman was that as the nature of a disease is understood more fully, the ability to define the role that nutrition plays in that disease process becomes more understandable. Another issue that came up repeatedly was the importance of defining nutritional status. Finally, consideration should be given to lessons learned from instances where nutritional status is well defined so they can be applied to other cases where nutritional status is not well defined. A related idea is the evolving understanding of what is considered a nutrient and the use of the term "essential nutrient" versus "conditionally essential nutrient." In several sessions, particularly around discussions about intestinal diseases, the focus is shifting from specific nutrient requirements to the broader concept of special dietary requirements or special dietary patterns. In addition, although advances in the tools used to study disease and nutrients are emerging, investigators and clinicians are still working with some old paradigms. In that sense, the use of these emerging tools as part of the repertoire of approaches for looking at special nutrient requirements could be explored, Schneeman observed.

The panel on future opportunities had four members. Susan Barr, Professor Emeritus of Food, Nutrition, and Health at the University of British Columbia, reflected on the workshop presentations from a perspective of the Dietary Reference Intakes (DRIs). Kristen D'Anci, Associate Director in the ECRI Institute's Evidence-based Practice Center and Health Technology Assessment group, provided remarks from the perspective of building clinical recommendations, evidence-based recommendations, and clinical guidelines. Timothy Morck, Founder and President of Spectrum Nutrition LLC, provided an industry perspective, and Virginia Stallings, Children's Hospital of Philadelphia, reflected on the workshop from her experience and perspective as a clinician.

PANEL DISCUSSION

Susan Barr

Barr posed the following key questions that the workshop presentations raised in relation to DRIs:

- Dietary requirements for what? People talk about "the requirement" for a nutrient, but in fact, Barr said, there are many requirements for any given nutrient, depending on the selected indicator of adequacy. This question has not been addressed explicitly in most of the DRIs[1] to date, but one example is vitamin A. The Estimated Average Requirement (EAR) for vitamin A intake in North America is based on adequate liver stores, and was set at 500 mcg/d for women and 625 mcg/d for men. The DRI report, however, includes a statement indicating that an EAR based on correction of impaired dark adap-

---

[1] For DRI values, see http://nationalacademies.org/HMD/Activities/Nutrition/SummaryDRIs/DRI-Tables.aspx (accessed June 6, 2018).

tation can be calculated as 300 mcg/d, and might be appropriate in less developed countries where vitamin A may not be as widely available (IOM, 2001, pp. 121–122).

- Requirement for what disease or health status? Are we looking for the requirement based on the same indicator of adequacy as was used in the apparently healthy population? Or would it be a different indicator of adequacy that is somehow adversely affected by the disease? Or an indication of reduction of disease progression that acts through altered nutrient needs?
- How are requirements and recommended intakes differentiated? Nutrient requirements are for individuals, but individual nutrient requirements do differ. It is very difficult for a clinician to determine an individual's requirement. It is possible to determine the average requirement (the EAR), but that meets the needs of only half the individuals in an age/sex group. If the goal is to cover the needs of almost everyone with a given disease, variability in requirements should be considered and recommended intakes identified.
- What happens to the requirement distribution in disease? It is possible that the presence of disease could simply shift the position of the requirement distribution by a fixed amount. However, it is much more likely that both the position and the variability of the requirement distribution may change due to factors such as disease severity, other comorbidities, inflammation, effective treatment, drugs, and surgery.
- What about upper levels of intake? A so-called safe range of intake has been established between the Recommended Dietary Allowance (RDA) and the Tolerable Upper Intake Level (UL), where both the risk of not getting enough and the potential risk of excess are low (see Figures 1-1 and 1-2). The magnitude of that safe range is not constant across nutrients, however. It is possible that the UL in a disease state might increase in parallel with the increase in the requirement, maintaining a similar "safe range" of intake. However, it is also possible that the UL in a disease state would not change if it were based on an adverse effect that was not affected by the disease state.
- How should competing risks be managed? If the disease shifts the requirement distribution to the right so that more is needed to achieve adequacy, a group of people with the disease would possibly be receiving levels above the UL, and that would place a proportion of that group of people at risk of adverse effects. How should those competing risks be managed?
- Is it possible to individualize? If sensitive, specific, non-invasively obtained, and inexpensive biomarkers were available, it might be

possible to titrate an individual's intake of the nutrient so that he or she could meet an individual requirement.

Kristen D'Anci

Clinical practice guidelines are statements that include recommendations to optimize patient care. They are informed by a systematic review of the evidence and assessment of the benefits and harms of alternative care options. D'Anci identified the following challenges in translating the research:

- Nutrition interventions are complex and must be considered in the context of the diet as a whole. Unlike with drug interventions, nutrients are not being given in a vacuum. People are eating, doing other things, and they may not be compliant with the intervention.
- Many of the disease states discussed at this workshop are rare. A small patient population has the additional complication of heterogeneity due to issues such as age, disease state, other factors in the diet and environment, and genetic makeup.
- The current evidence base is extremely limited. A systematic review that is done to support a guideline must be done in a way that facilitates decision making and should use a best-evidence approach, which could potentially include using evidence from case series and case reports. Such systematic reviews differ from those that limit their inclusion criteria to randomized controlled trials (RCTs), which are done to determine the causal link between an intervention and outcome. Once the systematic review is completed, the guideline panel works with the evidence and also considers many issues besides just the evidence itself, including the balance of benefits and harms, patient values and preferences, and other factors. The panel then uses all of these factors to make a recommendation.
- Determining how to assess the quality of the evidence is challenging. Grading of Recommendations Assessments, Development and Evaluation (GRADE) is a commonly used framework in guideline development. For much of the research described in this workshop, the quality of evidence may actually be graded up based on effect sizes, generalizability of the patient population, adequate ascertainment of exposures and outcomes, dose response, alternative explanations of causality, and length of follow-up.

D'Anci observed that a number of groups are considering new paradigms for determining adequacy of evidence, such as rethinking the concept that RCTs are the best designs and considering other rigorous study designs in supporting guidelines. Some groups are even considering ways of evaluating evidence from animal studies.

Timothy Morck

Morck reviewed the following ideas that emerged from the workshop from his perspective:

- It is important to document nutrient needs and establish therapeutic dose and composition, so that medical nutrition therapy for disease states can be standardized.
- The patient bears the burden of the disease. The more industry and researchers can accelerate the process of getting effective "therapeutic nutritional" products into the hands of patients who are already under the supervision of a doctor who has recommended them for their specific condition, the better the outcomes will be.
- The workshop has elevated the role of nutrition as a central part of cost-effective patient care. Many of the products that can be used in nutritional therapy can reduce symptoms and complications of diseases associated with nutritional imbalance, with a larger benefit–cost ratio compared to drugs that are being used to manage the disease. Such drugs, by design, may be relatively toxic, but seldom contribute to the body's healing or restorative processes, as do nutrients.
- A clear scientific process that is able to establish distinctive nutritional requirements in a disease state will promote the rapid development of an appropriate regulatory framework to guide industry in developing safe and efficacious products that benefit patients. Faster progress in identifying and validating appropriate nutritional biomarkers is imperative.
- How do we get solutions, now? The food industry and the scientific community are both full of good ideas, but it will be important to ensure that these nutritional innovations are consistent with clinical practice guidelines to modulate the disease progression, the severity of the disease, the side effects, or the interaction with drugs and treatment therapies to improve overall nutritional status.
- Decisions about regulating medical foods should consider the fact that medical foods require initial recommendation and ongoing supervision by health care professionals. This ensures proper monitoring of outcomes and continuous modifications of a particular intervention. Therefore, the level of evidence that is needed for medical food regulations could be different from the level of evi-

dence for other public health decisions that do not involve direct medical supervision.

Morck concluded his remarks by saying that the workshop highlighted the importance of efforts to increase the priority of funding for this arena of nutritional research.

Virginia Stallings

Stallings rounded out the panelist remarks with the following observations:

- Clinicians have little information and feel hamstrung in trying to use evidence-based decisions to guide them in caring for their patients.
- Clinical judgment is crucial in making clinical guidelines in the absence of robust evidence. Clinicians have the responsibility to keep moving the field forward and include the new thinking about study design, data collection, and evidence standards in clinical care.
- Until recently, the *Dietary Guidelines for Americans* and the DRI process have remained relatively silent on chronic disease issues. However, more than 50 percent of the adult population now has a chronic disease. This new paradigm needs considerable work when thinking about nutritional requirements and the DRIs.
- Clinicians are faced with the task of identifying a variety of clinical decisions and actions that might contribute to disease prevention or that might be useful in managing the disease or preventing progression. How does nutrition fit into those actions?
- The difference in nutritional needs between an acute illness event and those for an ongoing chronic illness presents a real clinical and research opportunity. Most clinicians think about nutrition in the setting of chronic diseases, but could clinicians use nutrition-related therapy in the emergency room to manage, for example, sickle cell pain crises?

OPEN DISCUSSION AND Q&A

Schneeman opened the discussion by referring back to the points made in the previous session (see Chapter 5) about various kinds of tensions, including those between the nutrient focus and the dietary focus, the genetic focus and the phenotypic focus, individuals and populations, final health outcomes and biomarkers in the pathway, and acute and chronic diseases. Such tensions can be used to advance scientific and clinical understanding by identifying the issues that need to be resolved in order to make progress.

Panelists responded that they were hopeful that the workshop would lead to action. They also concurred that much of the tension derives from a lack of understanding of what question is being asked, and time spent in dialogue would be beneficial.

Defining the Terms

Other tensions identified by the panelists related to defining terms (e.g., "nutrient" or "chronic disease") and to differences between the scientific approach and the clinician approach. The clinical principal of "do no harm" must be central to decisions about how to apply new evidence to clinical settings. An example of tensions or questions related to terminology is the need for a term that might encompass bioactives, such as phytonutrients, and other non-nutrient compounds so that they might be considered for inclusion in medical foods.

In terms of defining special dietary requirements, situations where patients have nutrient needs within the DRI range, but perhaps with a narrower range of tolerance, were raised. In this case, a way of defining "special" or "distinct" nutrient, would not mean a shift in the DRI distribution curve of requirement. This discussion led to the needed distinction between a recommendation for a group versus a recommendation for a specific individual. In the context of the DRI, some groups that might have distinct nutrient requirements, such as smokers and vitamin C or vegetarians and iron, have been considered. In the context of a disease state, if a person's tolerance of a nutrient is very low, that requires individual monitoring.

What Constitutes Sufficient Proof?

The panelists reflected on a question about what constitutes proof for a distinctive nutritional requirement, given the need by patients, clinicians, and industry to have a regulatory framework for nutritional therapy. Companies can create any medical foods, but clinicians need evidence of effectiveness for nutrients or other bioactive compounds. Schneeman stated that as the science has advanced because of better genetic and metabolic tools, nutrition requirements beyond those of inborn errors of metabolism are being considered.

Susan Barr was asked to comment on whether the DRI category of Adequate Intake (AI) could help address the dilemma of a limited evidence base. Barr replied that the AI has been a challenge in terms of determining what it really means and how to interpret intakes that are below the AI. Although healthy individuals who meet or exceed the AI for a nutrient can generally be assumed to meet their requirements, no assessment can be made when intakes are below the AI. Some of the AIs were set using median intakes of a healthy population. In this setting, half the population would have intakes below the AI, but the prevalence of inadequacy (i.e., not meeting one's requirement) could be extremely low. However, it is possible that for disease states for which the evidence base is limited, a different term could be identified.

CLOSING REMARKS

Paul Coates, National Institutes of Health

Coates commented on three concepts repeated throughout the workshop: evidence, uncertainty, and complexity. From his perspective, gathering the evidence to clarify requirements different from those for the general population is key. The evidence that a clinician intervention with a nutritional approach may make a difference in patient-reported outcomes and clinical outcomes is still insufficient. Biomarkers may be able to help provide the evidence to estimate the impact of an intervention on an outcome.

Entirely related to that evidence question is the issue of certainty or uncertainty. Past DRI efforts have acknowledged that uncertainty is associated with those values. The use of GRADE and other systems to assess the quality of intervention trials, observational studies, and animal studies would greatly help in assessing the uncertainty of estimates.

The third issue is complexity. Inborn errors of metabolism, in all of their complexity, are a harbinger of what is in the future as principles of nutritional management are translated from specific disease states to broader chronic disease indications.

Finally, innovations in identifying people at risk, developing strategies for assessing the impact of interventions, and analyzing data are all needed to be able to make recommendations in the context of increasing disease rates in populations.

Patricia Hansen, U.S. Food and Drug Administration

Hansen noted that the workshop cuts across the U.S. Food and Drug Administration's (FDA's) mission areas, including medical foods, foods for special dietary use, and even some specialized infant formulas; dietary supplements; and drugs as well. This is very important as FDA carries out its role in basing sound policies and regulations on sound, strong, and consensus science.

Hansen expressed her appreciation for the thoughtful presentations on a wide spectrum of diseases and the foundational presentations, which discussed how using lessons learned from the DRIs, both positive and negative, can be applied from those experiences to considering the role of nutrition in disease. She expressed hope for the workshop themes to stimulate the research and clinical community to fill these important gaps that will be essential in efforts to move forward with a modern framework that incorporates the best of science.

Caren Heller, Crohn's & Colitis Foundation

Heller stated that the Foundation welcomed the opportunity to support this workshop, because nutrition and diet are so important to patients with these diseases. Ways to support inflammatory bowel disease (IBD) patients within the arenas of both diet as therapy and diet to maintain nutritional health are challenging, particularly because so many are at risk of malnutrition.

In terms of diet as therapy, Heller said, it is clear that more science is needed to support interventions. In addition, regulatory and reimbursement hurdles make it difficult for patients to access enteral nutritional products. Heller noted that the Foundation is working with groups like the North American Society for Pediatric Gastroenterology, Hepatology, and Nutrition, and the American Gastrological Association, to engage on legislative acts to improve access. She highlighted other specific questions, such as what kind of study designs and scientific data would guide FDA in defining a more streamlined regulatory approval and affect reimbursement decisions and what research studies the Foundation can be engaged in to further the understanding of special nutritional requirements in IBD to facilitate the regulatory framework.

Chantal Martineau, Health Canada

Martineau explained that the Bureau of Nutritional Science at Health Canada has the responsibility to develop and update regulations related to foods for special dietary use. These include meal replacements, nutritional supplements, medical foods (e.g., enteral products), and products developed for low amino acid and low protein diets.

Gaining a better understanding of the evidence base available related to variations in nutritional requirements associated with various diseases and conditions is an important first step to potentially establish a framework for determining special nutrition requirements, she said, although much work still needs to be done.

In Canada, regulations for most foods used for special dietary use include detailed compositional requirements for micronutrients. Canada has minimum and maximum levels for macronutrients and vitamins and minerals, along with protein quality requirements, and these compositional provisions are very strict and based on requirements for the healthy population. Canada has initiated the process to review and update the regulations, as they were all established in the 1980s and 1990s, and Health Canada intends to consider the evidence presented at this workshop as it updates the regulations.

Sarah Ohlhorst, American Society for Nutrition

Ohlhorst described that in 2015, the American Society for Nutrition (ASN) brought together a working group, the Food for Health Initiative, with members from the academic community, nutrition and health organizations, patient groups, industry stakeholders, and many others to look at nutritional requirements for those living with disease or certain medical conditions from a nutrition science perspective.

A nutritional requirement to meet or restore desired health outcomes for one individual may vary quite drastically from that of another individual living with the same disease or medical condition, and so there are many considerations at play. More research is certainly needed to help elucidate the evidence base behind these special nutritional requirements so that next steps for a path forward can be determined. ASN plans to continue the dialogue and continue having these discussions with its Food for Health working group and with any other interested parties.

Alison Steiber, Academy of Nutrition and Dietetics

Steiber commented that the Academy of Nutrition and Dietetics (AND) practitioners care for individuals with many different diseases. AND has a major interest in understanding how nutrition can improve health outcomes, particularly for at-risk individuals and to work with those patients and their caregivers to help them understand their diet as well as to help them make a diet that is palatable and will meet their chronic disease needs. Echoing other speakers, Steiber stated that biomarkers for nutrients are needed that are rapid, feasible in clinical settings, and cost-effective. Practitioners must be given practical yet evidence-based guidelines on which they can look at macro- and micronutrients and dietary patterns for individuals living with disease states.

AND has recently completed both the scoping for evidence of nutrition requirements in cystic fibrosis and a very large evidence-based practice guideline project in collaboration with the National Kidney Foundation. Using the GRADE methodology, macronutrients have some moderate and high-level evidence recommendations. However, for micronutrient needs in the chronic kidney disease population at all stages, very few recommendations are above a low strength of evidence level.

Steiber noted that this process has helped to identify gaps in the evidence, but implementing recommendations is a challenge for practitioners. Finally, she emphasized that in lieu of good biomarkers, researchers could use (and document in the electronic medical records) nutrition-focused physical exams and composite nutrition diagnostic tools, such as subjective global assessment and malnutrition clinical characteristics, in their research across different states.

REFERENCE

IOM. 2001. *Dietary Reference Intakes for vitamin A, vitamin K, arsenic, boron, chromium, copper, iodine, iron, manganese, molybdenum, nickel, silicon, vanadium, and zinc.* Washington, DC: National Academy Press.

Appendix A

Workshop Agenda

**Examining Special Nutritional Requirements in Disease States:
A Workshop**

**Planning Committee on Examining
Special Nutritional Requirements in Disease States**

**April 2–3, 2018
National Academy of Sciences Building
Lecture Room
2101 Constitution Avenue, NW
Washington, DC**

Workshop Objectives

- Examine pathophysiological mechanisms by which specific diseases impact nutrient metabolism and nutrition status and whether this impact would result in nutrient requirements that differ from the Dietary Reference Intakes.
  - Explore the role of genetic variation in nutrition requirements.
  - Examine nutrient requirements in certain chronic conditions or acute phases for which emerging data suggest a contribution of nutrition status to disease outcomes. Consider the scientific evidence needed to establish such relationships and discuss principles about the relationship between nutrition requirements and specific diseases.

- o Explore how a disease state impacts nutrient metabolism and nutritional status and, conversely, how nutritional status impacts the disease state.
- Identify promising approaches and challenges to establishing a framework for determining special nutrient requirements related to managing disease states.

WORKSHOP DAY 1: APRIL 2, 2018, 8:30 AM–5:15 PM

7:30–8:30 AM   Registration

Session 1: Introduction of the Concepts and Context of the Workshop
Moderator: Barbara Schneeman, University of California, Davis

8:30   Origins of the Workshop
Barbara Schneeman, University of California, Davis, Planning Committee Chair

8:50   What Defines a Special Nutritional Requirement?
Patsy Brannon, Cornell University

9:10   The Underlying Biological Processes of Special Nutritional Requirements
Patrick Stover, Texas A&M AgriLife

9:30   Moderated Panel Discussion and Q&A

10:00   Break

Session 2: Addressing Nutrient Needs Due to Loss of Function in Genetic Diseases
Moderator: Erin MacLeod, Children's National Health System

10:20   Understanding the Basis of Nutritional Needs in Phenylketonuria
Denise Ney, University of Wisconsin–Madison

10:40   Nutritional Inadequacies in Mitochondrial-Associated Metabolic Disorders
Marni Falk, Children's Hospital of Philadelphia (via Zoom)

11:00   Contribution of Nutrients in Complex Inborn Errors of Metabolism: The Case of Methylmalonic Acidemia (MMA)
Charles Venditti, National Human Genome Research Institute, National Institutes of Health

11:20   Lessons Learned: What We Know About Nutrition
Management for Inborn Errors of Metabolism
Sue Berry, University of Minnesota

11:40   Moderated Panel Discussion and Q&A

12:00–1:00 PM   Lunch

Session 3: Disease-Induced Loss of Function and Tissue Regeneration
Moderator: Alex Kemper, Nationwide Children's Hospital

1:00   Examples of Gastrointestinal Dysfunction and
Malabsorption of Nutrients: Intestinal Failure
Chris Duggan, Boston Children's Hospital (via Zoom)

1:30   Examples of Gastrointestinal Dysfunction and
Malabsorption of Nutrients: Cystic Fibrosis
Sarah Jane Schwarzenberg, University of Minnesota
Masonic Children's Hospital

1:50   Nutritional Requirements for Inflammatory Bowel
Disease
Dale Lee, Seattle Children's Hospital

2:10   Blood–Brain Barrier Dysfunction and Resulting Brain
Nutrient Deficiencies
Martha Field, Cornell University

2:30   Macro- and Micronutrient Homeostasis in the Setting of
Chronic Kidney Disease
Alp Ikizler, Vanderbilt University

2:50   Moderated Panel Discussion and Q&A

3:15   Break

**Session 4: Disease-Induced Deficiency and Conditionally Essential
Nutrients in Disease**
*Moderator: Bernadette Marriott, Medical University of South
Carolina*

3:30   Arginine as an Example of a Conditionally Essential
Nutrient: Sickle Cell Anemia and Surgery
Claudia Morris, Emory University School of Medicine

3:50	Nutritional Needs in Hypermetabolic States: Burns, Cachexia, and Surgery
	Paul Wischmeyer, Duke University School of Medicine
	[NOTE: He did not speak at the workshop.]

4:10	Traumatic Brain Injury: Pathophysiological Mechanisms and Potential Nutrient Needs
	Angus Scrimgeour, U.S. Army Research Institute of Environmental Medicine

4:30	Metabolic Turnover, Inflammation, and Redistribution: Impact on Nutrient Requirements
	Jesse Gregory, University of Florida

| 4:50 | Moderated Panel Discussion and Q&A |

| 5:15 | Adjourn First Day |

WORKSHOP DAY 2: APRIL 3, 2018, 8:30 AM–1:00 PM

| 7:30–8:30 AM | Registration |

Session 5: Building the Evidence Base: Research Approaches for Nutrients in Disease States

Moderator: Alex Kemper, Nationwide Children's Hospital

8:30	Type and Strength of Evidence Needed for Determining Special Nutrient Requirements
	Amanda MacFarlane, Health Canada

8:50	Identification and Validation of Biomarkers in Disease States
	Patrick Stover, Texas A&M AgriLife

9:10	Innovative Causal Designs for Efficacy: What Type of Evidence Is Needed?
	Nicholas Schork, J. Craig Venter Institute

9:30	Examples of a Complex Disease
	• Inflammatory Bowel Disease
	Gary Wu, University of Pennsylvania
	• Cancer
	Steve Clinton, The Ohio State University

| 10:15 | Moderated Panel Discussion and Q&A |

| 10:45 | Break |

Session 6: Future Opportunities

Moderator: Barbara Schneeman, University of California, Davis

11:00   Principles Learned from Workshop Presentations
Barbara Schneeman, University of California, Davis

11:20   Panel Discussion
Susan Barr, University of British Columbia
Kristen D'Anci, ECRI Institute (via Zoom)
Tim Morck, Spectrum Nutrition LLC
Virginia A. Stallings, Children's Hospital of Philadelphia

12:30 PM   Sponsor Remarks
Paul Coates, National Institutes of Health
Patricia Hansen, U.S. Food and Drug Administration
Caren Heller, Crohn's & Colitis Foundation
Chantal Martineau, Health Canada
Sarah Ohlhorst, American Society for Nutrition
Alison Steiber, Academy of Nutrition and Dietetics

1:00   Meeting Adjourned

Appendix B

Speaker and Moderator Biographical Sketches

Susan I. Barr, Ph.D., is Professor Emeritus of Food, Nutrition, and Health at the University of British Columbia. Her research interests relate to how women's cognitions about food, eating, and body weight may have physiological implications for their health. She has also done work examining dietary practices and nutrient adequacy. Dr. Barr was involved in the development of the initial Dietary Reference Intakes (DRIs) as a member and Chair of the Subcommittee on Interpretation and Uses of DRIs, and subsequently served on the Committee on Development of Guiding Principles for the Inclusion of Chronic Disease Endpoints in Future Dietary Reference Intakes. She has also been a member of a number of Health Canada committees. Dr. Barr received her Ph.D. in human nutrition from the University of Minnesota and has received awards for teaching, research, and service.

Susan A. Berry, M.D., is Division Director for Genetics and Metabolism in the Department of Pediatrics at the University of Minnesota. She has been at the University of Minnesota since 1978, where she completed her residency in Pediatrics and was a fellow in Medical Genetics. She joined the staff of the Department in 1984 and is currently a Professor in the Departments of Pediatrics; Ophthalmology and Visual Neurosciences; and Genetics, Cell Biology, and Development. Dr. Berry's research focuses on long-term follow-up for newborn-screened conditions. As a nationally recognized geneticist and expert in inborn errors of metabolism, Dr. Berry sees both child and adult patients for genetic consultation at the

University of Minnesota Physicians Pediatric Specialty Clinic. She also attends the Pediatric and Adult Metabolic Clinics, providing care for children and adults with inborn errors of metabolism. She also offers her expertise for inpatient consultation and care. Dr. Berry is a member of the Minnesota Department of Health Newborn Screening Advisory Committee, the Society for Inherited Metabolic Disorders, and the American Society of Human Genetics, and she is a Fellow of the American Academy of Pediatrics and of the American College of Medical Genetics. Dr. Berry received her M.D. from the University of Kansas.

Patsy M. Brannon, Ph.D., R.D., is a Professor in the Division of Nutritional Sciences at Cornell University, where she has also served as Dean of the College of Human Ecology. Before moving to Cornell University, Dr. Brannon was Chair of the Department of Nutrition and Food Science, University of Maryland. She has also served as Visiting Professor at the Office of Dietary Supplements of the National Institutes of Health. Her research focus includes nutritional and metabolic regulation of gene expression, especially as relating to human development, the placenta, and exocrine pancreas. She was a member of the National Academies of Sciences, Engineering, and Medicine's Committee on Dietary Reference Intakes for Vitamin D and Calcium, and she is currently a member of the National Academies' Food and Nutrition Board. Dr. Brannon is a member of a number of professional and scientific associations and has served on the Executive Board of the American Society for Nutrition. She has received numerous awards, including the Pew Faculty Scholar in Nutrition award as well as the Centennial Laureate award from Florida State University. Dr. Brannon received her Ph.D. from Cornell University in nutritional biochemistry.

Steven K. Clinton, M.D., Ph.D., is a Professor in the Department of Internal Medicine, Division of Medical Oncology at The Ohio State University. He is the Program Leader for the Molecular Carcinogenesis and Chemoprevention Program of the Comprehensive Cancer Center and serves the James Cancer Hospital as Director of Prostate and Genitourinary Oncology. Dr. Clinton is a faculty member of the campus-wide Ohio State University Nutrition Graduate Program and is Co-Director of the Center for Advanced Functional Foods Research and Entrepreneurship. His research examines fundamental mechanisms underlying the development of cancer and studies novel prevention and therapeutic strategies in human clinical trials. His cancer research interests within nutritional sciences include the roles of energy intake, bioactive lipids, vitamin D, carotenoids, and other phytochemicals. Dr. Clinton received his M.D. from the

University of Illinois College of Medicine and his Ph.D. in Nutritional Sciences from the University of Illinois at Urbana-Champaign.

Kristen E. D'Anci, Ph.D., has more than 20 years of experience conducting and reporting scientific research in the biomedical fields, including drug abuse and nutrition. As an Associate Director in ECRI Institute's Evidence-based Practice Center (EPC) and Health Technology Assessment group, she performs and writes systematic reviews on topics such as medical treatments and behavioral health. Since joining ECRI, she has worked as Principal Investigator or Co-Investigator on clinical practice guidelines for the Department of Veterans Affairs/Department of Defense, the American College of Rheumatology, and an EPC report supporting upcoming guidelines from the National Institutes of Health's National Heart, Lung, and Blood Institute. Before her work at ECRI Institute, Dr. D'Anci was an Assistant Professor of Biopsychology at Salem State University in Salem, Massachusetts, and a biobehavioral researcher at Tufts University in Medford, Massachusetts. She completed two postdoctoral programs, one in Clinical Nutrition at Tufts University and one in Behavioral Pharmacology at Harvard University, and earned her doctorate in Experimental Psychology from Tufts University. In addition to her work at ECRI, she currently serves as Associate Editor for the journal *Nutrition Reviews* and she is a member of both the GRADE (Grading of Recommendations Assessment, Development and Evaluation) Working Group and the Guidelines International Network.

Christopher Duggan, M.D., M.P.H., is a Professor in the Departments of Nutrition and Global Health and Population at the Harvard T.H. Chan School of Public Health. He is also Professor of Pediatrics at Harvard Medical School and Director of the Center for Nutrition at the Boston Children's Hospital. His major research interests include the nutritional management of acute and persistent diarrhea, micronutrient trials in developing countries to prevent diarrhea and respiratory infections, the definition of biomarkers of environmental enteric dysfunction, and general aspects of energy and protein metabolism in catabolic diseases. He has completed studies in both developing and industrialized countries on the micronutrient status of children, including those with cystic fibrosis, malaria, undernutrition, and intestinal failure. Dr. Duggan has twice received the Physician Nutrition Specialist Award from the American Society of Nutrition, was the 2015 recipient of the Fomon Nutrition Award from the American Academy of Pediatrics, and has been a visiting professor in China, India, Tanzania, and many other countries. He received his M.D. from the Johns Hopkins University School of Medicine and his M.P.H. from the Harvard T.H. Chan School of Public Health.

Marni J. Falk, M.D., is Executive Director of the Mitochondrial Medicine Frontier Program at the Children's Hospital of Philadelphia (CHOP) and Associate Professor in the Division of Human Genetics within the Department of Pediatrics at the University of Pennsylvania Perelman School of Medicine. She works to improve diagnostic approaches and genomic resources for mitochondrial disease, including organization of a global Mitochondrial Disease Sequence Data Resource consortium. Dr. Falk is also the Principal Investigator of a translational research laboratory group at CHOP that investigates the causes and global metabolic consequences of mitochondrial disease, as well as targeted therapies, in *Caenorhabditis elegans*, zebrafish, mouse, and human tissue models of genetic-based respiratory chain dysfunction. She also directs multiple clinical treatment trials in mitochondrial disease patients and she has authored more than 90 publications in the areas of human genetics and mitochondrial disease. Dr. Falk also directs the CHOP/University of Pennsylvania Mitochondria Research Affinity Group, which has 250 participants. She is Chair of the Scientific and Medical Advisory Board and serves on the Board of Trustees of the United Mitochondrial Disease Foundation. She is a founding member of the CHOP Center for Mitochondrial and Epigenomic Medicine and is the CHOP-site Principal Investigator of the North American Mitochondrial Disease Consortium. She is a member of the Mitochondrial Medicine Society, Society for Pediatric Research, Society for Inherited Metabolic Disease, American Society of Human Genetics, and American College of Medical Genetics and Genomics, and is an elected member of the University of Pennsylvania John Morgan Society, Interurban Clinical Club, and American Society of Clinical Investigators. Dr. Falk received her M.D. from the George Washington University School of Medicine.

Martha S. Field, Ph.D., is an Assistant Professor in the Division of Nutritional Sciences at Cornell University. Her research focuses on understanding the complexity of gene–gene, gene–nutrient, and gene–nutrient–environment interactions that affect cellular metabolism and on the biochemical mechanisms whereby perturbations in metabolism affect human health and disease. Impaired folate-dependent one-carbon metabolism is associated with adverse physiological outcomes that include certain cancers, cardiovascular disease, neurological impairments, and birth defects. Dr. Field uses several in vitro and in vivo model systems to study the mechanisms that underlie physiological outcomes associated with perturbed one-carbon metabolism. More specifically, she is interested in the contributions of folate nutrition and enzyme localization in supporting mitochondrial DNA precursor synthesis, with a focus on understanding how folate nutrition affects mitochondrial DNA integrity and pathogenesis of metabolic diseases such as mitochondrial DNA depletion syndromes, chronic disease, and age-related decline in mito-chondrial function. Recently, her research has focused on the metabolism of erythritol, which is a product of the pentose phosphate pathway and which has emerged as a biomarker of weight gain and adiposity in young adults. Dr. Field received her Ph.D. in biochemistry and molecular and cell biology from Cornell University.

Jesse F. Gregory, Ph.D., is a Professor of Food Science and Human Nutri-tion at the University of Florida. The focus of his research encompasses basic aspects of B vitamins in human nutrition and metabolism in health and disease. He has extensive research experience in mammalian vitamin metabolism, including folate and vitamin B6 analysis, chemistry, bioavail-ability, and metabolic function using in vivo studies with animal, cell, and human protocols. His research group has extensive experience with studies of folate and one-carbon metabolism, various global and targeted metabolomic methods, and stable isotopic tracer kinetic techniques to assess metabolic function and fluxes in humans. Dr. Gregory is Associate Editor of *The Journal of Nutrition* and was elected as a Fellow of the Ameri-can Society for Nutrition in 2016. Dr. Gregory received his Ph.D. in food science and human nutrition from Michigan State University.

T. Alp Ikizler, M.D., is the Catherine McLaughlin Hakim Chair in Vascu-lar Biology and Professor of Medicine at the Vanderbilt University School of Medicine (VUSM) in Nashville, Tennessee. He is Associate Director of the Division of Nephrology, a member of the American Society of Clini-cal Investigation (ASCI) and a member of ASCI Advocacy Committee. Dr. Ikizler's clinical interests and expertise are focused on the care of patients with chronic kidney disease, end-stage renal disease on maintenance dialysis, and acute kidney injury. Dr. Ikizler was the Medical Director and Chief Executive Officer of the Vanderbilt University Medical Center Out-patient Dialysis unit between 2000 and 2012. He has significant research and clinical interest in nutritional and metabolic aspects of acute and chronic disease states. As a clinical investigator focused on mechanisms of disease and patient-related outcomes, he is the Principal Investigator of a number of ongoing studies aimed at improving the outcomes and quality of life in patient populations ranging from early kidney disease to patients on maintenance dialysis and patients with acute kidney injury. He is cur-rently an Associate Editor for *Kidney International* and is Co-Editor of the *Handbook of Nutrition in Kidney Disease.* Previously he served as President of the International Society of Renal Nutrition and Metabolism, Associate Editor of the *Journal of the American Society of Nephrology,* Director of the Master of Science in Clinical Investigation Program at VUSM, and mem-ber and Chair of the American Board of Internal Medicine Nephrology

Test Writing Committee. He is the recipient of National Kidney Foundation Joel Kopple Award and the International Society of Renal Nutrition and Metabolism Thomas Addis Award. He has published more than 280 original articles, 50 editorial reviews, and 20 book chapters. Dr. Ikizler received his M.D. from the Istanbul University Faculty of Medicine.

Alex R. Kemper, M.D., is a board-certified pediatrician and Chief of the Division of Ambulatory Pediatrics at the Nationwide Children's Hospital, Columbus, Ohio. Dr. Kemper's clinical and research interests include improving the quality of care that children receive by strengthening the linkages between primary care, specialty care, and public health services. He has studied a wide array of preventive services, including the prevention of amblyopia, the early detection and treatment of lead poisoning, and newborn screening. Dr. Kemper joined the U.S. Preventive Services Task Force in January 2014. Dr. Kemper is Deputy Editor of *Pediatrics*, the leading journal in the nation covering issues of child health. He is also a member of many organizations and societies, including the American Academy of Pediatrics, the Academic Pediatric Association, the American Pediatric Society, and the Society for Pediatric Research. He directs the Condition Review Workgroup for the Secretary of Health and Human Services' Advisory Committee on Heritable Disorders in Newborns and Children, which makes evidence-based recommendations about conditions that should be recommended for inclusion in State newborn screening panels. Dr. Kemper also works with Bright Futures to develop an evidence-based process of making recommendations for services that should be included as part of routine pediatric preventive care. Dr. Kemper received a B.S.E. from Johns Hopkins University. He completed an M.P.H. in epidemiology and an M.S. in biomedical engineering, focusing on medical informatics, at the University of North Carolina. Dr. Kemper earned his M.D. from the Duke University Medical School, where he completed a pediatric internship and residency. He also completed a fellowship in health services research and a preventive medicine residency at the University of North Carolina.

Dale Lee, M.D., is an Assistant Professor of Pediatrics at the Seattle Children's Hospital at the University of Washington. He is the Chair of the Hospital Nutrition Committee and Director of the Celiac Disease Program. Dr. Lee is dual fellowship trained in Pediatric Gastroenterology and Nutrition from the Children's Hospital of Philadelphia and the University of Pennsylvania. In addition, he is trained in clinical epidemiology. Dr. Lee is an organizer for a multidisciplinary symposium on a "Food Systems Approach to Gut Health" with the Department of Food Science at The Pennsylvania State University. He is a current scholar in the Clinical

Research Scholar's Program at the Seattle Children's Hospital studying dietary therapy for inflammatory bowel disease (IBD) as well as studying the role of dietary exposures in IBD pathogenesis. Dr. Lee's research program incorporates a multidisciplinary approach, including clinical gastroenterology, clinical nutrition, food science, plant science, and nutrition epidemiology. Dr. Lee received his M.S. in clinical epidemiology from the University of Pennsylvania and his M.D. from The University of Texas Southwestern Medical School.

Amanda MacFarlane, Ph.D., is a Research Scientist and Head of the Micronutrient Research Section in the Nutrition Research Division at Health Canada. She is an Adjunct Professor in the Department of Biochemistry, Microbiology, and Immunology at the University of Ottawa and the Department of Biology at Carleton University. She received her Ph.D. in Biochemistry in 2004 at the University of Ottawa, for which she won the 2003 Ron Oelbaum Award for an Outstanding Canadian Research Scientist younger than age 35 years from the Juvenile Diabetes Research Foundation. She did her postdoctoral research with Dr. Patrick Stover at Cornell University, where she examined the effect of altered folate metabolism on genome stability and gene expression in models of colon cancer. She joined Health Canada in 2008 where she examines the impact of maternal and paternal folate intake on germline genomic and epigenomic stability, and its effect on offspring health and disease. She also uses national health survey data to identify the socioeconomic, dietary, and genetic determinants of folate and B vitamin status of Canadians. She is the Canadian lead and Chair of the Joint Canada–U.S. Dietary Reference Intakes Working Group. She was the Project Co-Director for the expert panel and workshop "Options for Addressing Consideration of Chronic Disease Endpoints for Dietary Reference Intakes (DRIs)."

Erin MacLeod, Ph.D., is Director of Metabolic Nutrition in the Division of Genetics and Metabolism at the Children's National Health System in Washington, DC. In her current position Dr. MacLeod is part of an experienced clinical team that manages more than 400 patients with inborn errors of metabolism and participates in a variety of clinical research projects. Her primary research focus has been the nutritional management of phenylketonuria (PKU). She participated in the clinical trials for glycomacropeptide and conducted a study to examine the change in phenylalanine tolerance in adults with PKU. She received her Ph.D. from the University of Wisconsin–Madison.

Bernadette Marriott, Ph.D., holds the positions of Professor, Division of Gastroenterology and Hepatology, Department of Medicine, and Professor, Military Division, Department of Psychiatry and Behavioral Sciences, Medical University of South Carolina. Dr. Marriott has 40 years of experience in the fields of nutrition, psychology, and comparative medicine with expertise in diet, nutrition, and chronic disease. Dr. Marriott has worked in scientific settings in the federal government, universities, and foundations. Former positions include founding Director of the Office of Dietary Supplements, National Institutes of Health (NIH); Associate Director, the National Academies' Food and Nutrition Board; Vice President, Research Triangle Institute International; and Research Vice Provost and Graduate Dean, Northern Arizona University. Her research has focused on clinical trials and nutritional epidemiology studies involving diet and health. She is currently leading or has recently led research projects funded by the U.S. Army, Department of Defense, NIH, U.S. Department of Agriculture, industry, and foundations. Ongoing and recent research has assessed the use of added sugar and sugar-sweetened beverages in the United States and the impact of fatty acid supplementation on cognitive performance under stress and measures of mental health status among military personnel and veterans and nonveterans at risk of suicide. She has published extensively, has been on a number of national committees, and university and nonprofit scientific advisory boards, and is a frequent speaker on diet, dietary supplements, and health. Dr. Marriott is currently a member of the National Academies' Food and Nutrition Board and was elected a Fellow of the American Society for Nutrition in 2016. She has a B.Sc. in biology/immunology from Bucknell University, a Ph.D. in psychology from King's College, University of Aberdeen, Scotland, and postgraduate training in trace mineral nutrition, comparative medicine, and advanced statistics.

Timothy A. Morck, Ph.D., is the Founder and President of Spectrum Nutrition, LLC, a consulting firm that provides expertise in nutrition-related basic/clinical research, product development, regulatory and public policy, and global scientific affairs. Dr. Morck's career includes clinical nutrition practice, research, and medical school faculty appointments (University of Kansas Medical Center; Eastern Virginia Medical School; and Veterans Affairs Medical Center, Hampton, Virginia), scientific association management (International Life Sciences Institute [ILSI]-North America), entrepreneurial personalized nutrition start-ups (MenuDirect Corp. and DSM Personalized Nutrition), and executive and senior management positions at several global food, nutrition, and pharmaceutical companies, including The Dannon Company, Mead Johnson Nutritionals, Abbott Nutrition, Nestlé Health Science, and Nestlé Corporate Affairs. His unique multidisciplinary perspective integrates scientific affairs and marketing to achieve business objectives, with a passion for personalized approaches that improve nutrition, health, and wellness for individuals, patients, and society. The interplay between the legal, scientific, and regulatory framework surrounding medical foods has been a particular focus for him. He received M.S. and Ph.D. degrees in nutrition (biochemistry and physiology minors) from Cornell University.

Claudia R. Morris, M.D., FAAP, is an Associate Professor of Pediatrics and Emergency Medicine at the Emory University School of Medicine. She is also a pediatric emergency medicine attending physician at Children's Healthcare of Atlanta. Dr. Morris has been involved in sickle cell disease (SCD) research for more than 20 years, has a history of the National Institutes of Health and the U.S. Food and Drug Administration/R01 and industry-sponsored funding, and has led several single and multi-center trials. She has a special interest in translational research that targets inflammation and oxidative stress. From the start of her career, Dr. Morris's research endeavors have focused on nutritional interventions based on specific metabolic pathways that cross disease disciplines, identifying alterations in the arginine metabolome in SCD, thalassemia, asthma, and pulmonary hypertension. She also published the first randomized, blinded, placebo-controlled trial of arginine therapy to treat pain in children with SCD. Dr. Morris's efforts have always encompassed an integrative approach to the practice of medicine. She is a firm believer in nutrition as medicine, and appreciates the growing need to address distinctive nutritional requirements provoked by some acute and chronic illnesses, with SCD as an ideal paradigm. Dr. Morris received her M.D. from Eastern Virginia Medical School.

Denise Ney, Ph.D., is a Professor of Nutritional Sciences and Affiliate Faculty Waisman Center, University of Wisconsin–Madison. Throughout her 30-year career as a faculty member at the University of Wisconsin–Madison, Dr. Ney has used surgical and genetic animal models where dietary manipulation was a primary variable to test a specific hypothesis. This research has resulted in translation of her research findings to humans for the treatment of short bowel syndrome and since 2003, the genetic disorder phenylketonuria (PKU). Her current research program to improve the nutritional management of PKU has resulted in a new paradigm for the PKU diet using glycomacropeptide medical foods. Dr. Ney is the 2015 recipient of the Mary Swartz Rose Senior Investigator Award from the American Society for Nutrition. She received her Ph.D. in nutrition sciences from the University of California, Davis.

Barbara O. Schneeman, Ph.D., served as the Higher Education Coordinator at the U.S. Agency for International Development from 2015–2016. From 2004 to 2013 she was the Director of the Office of Nutrition, Labeling, and Dietary Supplements at the U.S. Food and Drug Administration (FDA). In that position, she oversaw the development of policy and regulations for dietary supplements, labeling, food standards, infant formula, and medical foods and served as U.S. delegate to two Codex committees (Food Labeling and Nutrition and Foods for Special Dietary Uses). From 1976–2004, she was a member of the nutrition faculty at the University of California, Davis (UC Davis), and is currently emerita professor of nutrition. At UC Davis she served in several administrative roles, including Chair of the Department of Nutrition, Dean of the College of Agricultural and Environmental Sciences, and Associate Vice Provost for University Outreach. She has been a visiting scientist at the University of California, San Francisco, and Assistant Administrator for Nutrition in the Agricultural Research Service of the U.S. Department of Agriculture (USDA). Professional activities include participation in Dietary Guidelines Advisory Committees; being a past member of the National Academies' Food and Nutrition Board; and serving as a member of committees for the National Academies, USDA, the Food and Agriculture Organization, the World Health Organization, the American Society for Nutrition, and the Institute of Food Technologists. She has been Associate Editor for the *Journal of Nutrition* and on several editorial boards, including *Nutrition Reviews*, *Journal of Nutrition*, and *Journal of Food Science*. Her professional honors include Fellow of the American Society of Nutrition, Fellow of the American Association for the Advancement of Science, the Carl Fellers Award from the Institute of Food Technologists, the FDA Commissioner's Special Citation and the Harvey W. Wiley Medal, the FDA Merit Award, the Samuel Cate Prescott Award for research, Future Leader Award, and several honorary lectureships. She is recognized for her work on dietary fiber, gastrointestinal function, development and use of food-based dietary guidelines, and policy development in food and nutrition. She received her Ph.D. in nutrition from the University of California, Berkeley.

Nicholas J. Schork, Ph.D., is Distinguished Professor of Quantitative Medicine at the Translational Genomics Research Institute in Phoenix, Arizona; Professor and Director of Human Biology at the J. Craig Venter Institute (JCVI) in La Jolla, California; and an Adjunct Professor of Psychiatry and Family Medicine and Public Health (Division of Biostatistics) at the University of California, San Diego, in La Jolla, California. Before joining JCVI, Dr. Schork held faculty positions at The Scripps Research Institute, the Scripps Translational Science Institute, and Case Western Reserve University. Dr. Schork's interests and expertise are in quantitative human biomedical science and integrated approaches to complex biological and medical problems. He has published more than 500 scientific articles and book chapters that consider novel data analysis methodology, study designs, and applications. He has also mentored more than 75 graduate student and postdoctoral fellows, has 8 patents, and has helped establish 10 different companies in the biomedical science and applications. A member of several scientific journal editorial boards, Dr. Schork is a frequent participant in National Institutes of Health (NIH)-related steering committees and review boards. He is director of the quantitative components of a number of national research consortia, including the NIH-sponsored Longevity Consortium and the National Institute of Mental Health–sponsored Bipolar Consortium. Dr. Schork earned his M.A. in philosophy, M.A. in statistics, and Ph.D. in epidemiology from the University of Michigan, Ann Arbor.

Sarah Jane Schwarzenberg, M.D., is currently an Associate Professor in the Department of Pediatrics and the Chief of Pediatric Gastroenterology, Hepatology, and Nutrition at the University of Minnesota Masonic Children's Hospital. Dr. Schwarzenberg's initial research was in the area of hepatic gene regulation during inflammation. She now focuses on clinical research in cystic fibrosis–associated gastrointestinal disease and nutrition and in chronic pancreatitis in childhood. She is a member of the Committee on Nutrition of the American Academy of Pediatrics. Dr. Schwarzenberg is the 2017 recipient of the Murray Davidson Award from the American Academy of Pediatrics Section on Gastroenterology, Hepatology, and Nutrition. She received her M.D. from the University of Tennessee Medical School.

Angus Scrimgeour, Ph.D., is a nutritional biochemist in the Military Nutrition Division at the U.S. Army Research Institute of Environmental Medicine, in Natick, Massachusetts. He received his M.Sc. in physiology and sports medicine from the University of Cape Town, South Africa, and his Ph.D. in cell and molecular biology from the University of Vermont. He has more than 15 years of experience developing animal models of human disease to validate nutritional countermeasures. Mild traumatic brain injury (mTBI) has become the signature injury in the current war(s) and to address this problem, Dr. Scrimgeour has developed nutritional interventions that increase resiliency to neurotrauma in animal models. Initial efforts have involved working with the Royal Dutch Military, studying the effects of explosive blast in rats on marginally zinc-deficient diets, and reporting on the cognitive deficits associated with mild-to-moderate TBI. Current research efforts use both blast and non-blast models to induce mTBI in rats, and then using anti-inflammatory, neuroprotectant food-supplements (containing omega-3, vitamin D, and/or zinc) to increase resiliency to the effects of neurotrauma. In 2017, this work effort was expanded to use similar diets in pre-clinical models of posttraumatic stress disorder.

Virginia A. Stallings, M.D., is the Jean A. Cortner Endowed Chair in Pediatric Gastroenterology, Professor of Pediatrics and Nutrition, and Director of the Nutrition Center at the Children's Hospital of Philadelphia. Her research interests include pediatric nutrition, evaluation of dietary intake and energy expenditure, and nutrition-related chronic disease. Dr. Stallings has served on several National Academies committees, including the Committee on Food Allergies: Global Burden, Causes, Treatment, Prevention, and Public Policy; the Committee on Nutrition Standards for National School Lunch and Breakfast Programs; the Committee on Nutrition Services for Medicare Beneficiaries; the Committee on the Scientific Basis for Dietary Risk Eligibility Criteria for WIC (Special Supplemental Nutrition Program for Women, Infants, and Children) Programs; the Committee to Review the WIC Food Packages; and the Committee to Review Child and Adult Care Food Program Meal Requirements. She is a former member and Co-Vice Chair (2000–2002) of the National Academies' Food and Nutrition Board. Dr. Stallings is board certified in pediatrics and clinical nutrition. She received the Fomon Nutrition Award from the American Academy of Pediatrics. Dr. Stallings earned an M.S. in human nutrition and biochemistry from Cornell University and an M.D. from the University of Alabama at Birmingham School of Medicine. She is a member of the National Academy of Medicine.

Patrick J. Stover, Ph.D., is Vice Chancellor and Dean for Agriculture and Life Sciences at Texas A&M AgriLife. He previously served as the Director of the Division of Nutritional Sciences at Cornell University. He is also Director of the World Health Organization Collaborating Centre on Implementation Research in Nutrition and Global Policy at Cornell University and past President of the American Society for Nutritional Sciences. Dr. Stover's research interests focus on the biochemical, genetic, and epigenetic mechanisms that underlie the relationships between folic acid and human pathologies, including neural tube defects and other developmental anomalies, cardiovascular disease, and cancer. Specific interests include the regulation of folate-mediated one-carbon metabolism and cellular methylation reactions, molecular basis of the fetal origins hypothesis, development of mouse models to elucidate mechanisms of folate-related pathologies, and nuclear one-carbon metabolism. In 2016, he was elected as a member of the National Academy of Sciences, and in 2014 was elected as a Fellow of the American Association for the Advancement of Science. In 2014, he received the State University of New York Chancellor's Award for Excellence in Scholarship and Creative Activities, the Osborne and Mendel Award for outstanding recent basic research accomplishments in nutrition from the American Society for Nutrition, and a MERIT award from the National Institute of Diabetes and

Digestive and Kidney Diseases. In 1996, he received the Presidential Early Career Award for Scientists and Engineers, the highest honor bestowed by the U.S. government on outstanding scientists and engineers beginning their independent careers. He has been selected as an Outstanding Educator four times by Cornell Merrill Presidential Scholars. Dr. Stover served two terms on the National Academies' Food and Nutrition Board and he served on the Board's Nutrigenomics Workshop Planning Group. Dr. Stover received his Ph.D. in biochemistry and molecular biophysics from the Medical College of Virginia.

David L. Suskind, M.D., is a Professor of Pediatrics in the Division of Gastroenterology at the University of Washington in Seattle. He is a pediatric gastroenterologist working within a tertiary care center at Seattle Children's Hospital. His research has focused on the effect of the fecal microbial transplant and diet on inflammatory bowel disease (IBD), both of which affect the fecal microbiome. Dr. Suskind has conducted studies on the clinical, laboratory, and microbiome changes that occur after fecal microbial transplantation as well as on nutritional treatment approaches in IBD. His research on the specific carbohydrate diet in IBD has shown that patients with active Crohn's disease and ulcerative colitis can go into clinical and biochemical remission with diet alone. His studies also examine the impact of diet on fecal microbiome composition. Clinically, he has focused his work within the Seattle Children's Hospital IBD center, where his mission is to improve the quality of care and clinical outcomes for patients with IBD by focusing on the patient and not just their disease. Dr. Suskind received his M.D. from the Louisiana State University Medical School.

Charles P. Venditti, M.D., Ph.D., is Head of the Organic Acid Research Section and Senior Investigator of the National Human Genome Research Institute at the National Institutes of Health (NIH). He is also an attending physician at the Mark O. Hatfield Clinical Center at NIH, where he has initiated a translational research program to study the natural history and clinical phenotype(s) of the hereditary methylmalonic acidemias (MMA) and cobalamin metabolic disorders. The clinical research studies are paralleled by laboratory investigations that have focused on the development of experimental systems to study the genetics, genomics, and biochemistry of organic acid metabolism in model organisms, including roundworms, mice, and zebrafish. Using a translational research approach, Dr. Venditti and his colleagues have published a number of papers that connect disease pathophysiology in MMA to mitochondrial dysfunction and prove the efficacy of gene therapy as a treatment for both MMA and propionic acidemia. Dr. Venditti was the 2009 recipient of a Presidential Early Career Award for Scientists and Engineers. Other awards include selection as an Outstanding New Investigator from the American Society of Gene and Cell Therapy in 2010 and election into the American Society of Clinical Investigation in 2012. Dr. Venditti received his M.D. and Ph.D. from The Pennsylvania State University.

Gary D. Wu, M.D., is the inaugural Ferdinand G. Weisbrod Professor in Gastroenterology at the Perelman School of Medicine, University of Pennsylvania. He is the Associate Chief for Research in the Division of Gastroenterology; Co-Director of the Penn-Children's Hospital of Philadelphia (CHOP) Microbiome Program; Associate Director of the Joint Penn-CHOP Center for Digestive, Liver, and Pancreatic Medicine; and the Associate Director of the Center for Molecular Studies in Digestive and Liver Disease in which he is the Director of its Molecular Biology Core. As a physician-scientist, Dr. Wu's laboratory focuses primarily on multidisciplinary team research in the gut microbiome to translate basic research at the wet bench into the clinical setting. Dr. Wu's research into the gut microbiome began nearly a decade ago with projects focused on the impact of diet on the composition of the gut microbiota initially funded by the National Institutes of Health's (NIH's) Human Microbiome Project. Dr. Wu co-directs a number of NIH-funded projects, including a study examining the association of the gut microbiome with its metabolome and their correlations with the development of rapid growth and childhood obesity in a large longitudinal prospective cohort of children as well as the effects of chronic kidney disease on the gut microbiome and its metabolome. Dr. Wu's laboratory is also investigating the co-metabolism of ammonia between the host and its microbiome through the hydrolysis of host urea by gut microbiota urease activity. To translate this technology into the clinical arena, he is leading a collaboration among the University of Pennsylvania, CHOP, and an industry partner, in a multidisciplinary effort to develop a microbiota-based therapy for patients with inborn errors of metabolism. Dr. Wu received his M.D. from Northwestern University Medical School.